Face Everything & Rise

Kelsey Walker

Dedication

For Hope, our baby in the clouds but always in our hearts.

For Christopher, my sweetheart and my forever Phil-Phling.

For Cayden and Ember, my lights in the darkness.

TABLE OF CONTENTS

My toes curled and uncurled in the cool sand. No, I was not on a beach, somewhere warm and celebratory. I was sitting on the bank of a gross old reservoir, a mile or two east of Cold Beer New Mexico. I am alone. I watched a storm swirl and build behind distant mountains. I breathed in the fishy smell of the reservoir. While it was no charm to the senses, it was a touchpoint for me. Where ex-boyfriends and I had laid under the stars, I sunbathed with friends and even punched an asshole in the face. Where laughter still lived in the win.

Positive. The first two tests were barely positive and what I told my friend was inconclusive. But the third was glaringly positive.

Fuck

I was also painfully single. The father had dumped me months earlier but was gracious enough to keep me as a side piece. So, here I was!

Fuck

The storm finally swelled past the mountains and had darkened the sky. The thunder started to rumble low and the lightning danced closer. It was the first time I had answered the thunder.

I lept to my feet and screamed.

CRACK!

The thunder bellowed back. I clenched my fists, gathered the dry, New Mexico air in my lungs and burst forth a scream that broke open my soul. I was scared, furious, and grieved. My long, black hair moved with the harsh wind and whipped my face.

I raised my fists, took one more step forward, and swung them to my sides while I screamed. It was my way of meeting nature with my defiance, strength, and fear.

I was fierce like a warrior and determined. Lightning shrieked across the sky. This is the first time I was meeting this woman—wild and untamed—a force to be reckoned with.

HOPE

[PART 1]

CHAPTER 1

The same day when I finally got the promotion that I had worked so hard for, I also found out I was pregnant. We went to Perkins that night to celebrate my promotion and stopped by Walmart to pick up a few things, including a pregnancy test, on the way home. We had been trying for another baby for months with no luck. So, what were the chances of us finding out that we were pregnant? Especially the very day I got a promotion. The answer was quite simply—our luck. You see, our luck was getting pregnant while we were already pregnant. This happens with one in two million babies. This is what happened with our son Cayden and a pregnancy we had lost. Our son Cayden was also born with bilateral clubbed feet—a birth condition that affects one child in a thousand.

My husband, Chris, and I went to the same elementary school together, our brothers had the same Scoutmaster and I often went to his house for haunted trail rides, but in fifth grade my family relocated to Chicago. I did not meet Christopher until we met unexpectedly, about ten years later, when I was working at Philmont Scout Ranch in Cimarron, New Mexico. Hundreds of miles from Chicago, hundreds of miles from Kansas City, I sat on a rock waiting for the bus to come to the "turn-around," which was Philmont-ease for a mountain access point. It was hot and I waited for four hours under the New Mexican sun before I saw a group of rangers I had recognized. I had called headquarters to inquire about the bus but had been hung up on. Twice! I walked over to the group of rangers and told them about my conversations with logistics. They relayed that they were waiting for their friend to pick them up and that I could have a ride if I wanted. A group of dining hall staff came over the hill. They too needed the bus so we all waited.

A dark blue single cab truck drove into the turn around. We loaded our gear and the gentlemen into the bed of the truck and they were gracious enough to let myself and the other female staffer sit in the cab of the truck. I sat in the middle seat. The girl next to me struck up a conversation about being from Missouri with the boy driving the truck. I had seen him around camp before but did not know his name. They asked each other which high school they went to and when he said Lee's Summit

North, he immediately caught my attention and I turned my face to see him.

"Did you go to Hazel Grove?"

His head whipped to face mine, "How do you know about Hazel Grove, you're from Chicago?"

I explained how my dad got a promotion moving us away from Lee's Summit when we were little. The rest was history.

What were the chances of two perfect strangers meeting each other in a remote mountain terrain? It was our luck.

Unfortunately, it was also our luck that our daughter Hope would be extremely sick.

It was a fast move—two weeks—from the time I got the promotion offer to moving from Jefferson City, Missouri to Salina, Kansas. Everything went as smoothly as it could. Volunteers and Mr. Dennis came to help unload the moving truck, and I simply blamed my back on my inability to lift things out of the truck. It was in August when our family had spent all weekend with my coworkers on the Council Grove Lake, that we celebrated that we were pregnant.

It was Tuesday and I had spent the morning talking to youth and getting them excited to go camping, fishing, and rock climbing with the coolest club in town. I had an important doctor appointment before more talks with schools in the afternoon. It was the day when we would get to see a sonogram of our baby and find out if we were having a boy or a girl! I waited in the lobby, texting Christopher who was still on his way to the appointment about sanding down the old crib since Cayden had scratched it up with his braces from clubbed feet. We hoped that this baby would not have clubbed feet like their brother. It was so hard on Cayden growing up with the hip-to-toe casts and then ponseti braces until last May. I was also texting my mom, who insisted on throwing me a gender reveal with the theme "bows or arrows." I was enjoying the attention.

Christopher arrived and we walked back to the ultrasound room. It was warm and dim-lit. I laid back on the table and pulled my shirt up. The ultrasound technician squirted goo onto my belly from a bottle and ran the transponder over my abdomen. Christopher and I chatted while looking at our baby on the screen but eventually stopped when we noticed the silence of the ultrasound technician. She had been friendly before but she briskly asked me how far along I was to which I responded eighteen weeks. She told us there was no way I was eighteen weeks, as the baby she was measuring was clearly only big enough to be sixteen weeks. Also, the baby had its legs crossed so she could not even see the gender.

I furrowed my brow in confusion and asked, "Is everything healthy though?"

She flatly responded to my question saying, "The doctor will go over your results with you."

An icy feeling crept up my spine and made my hair stand at the end. But I continued to nervously chatter with Christopher in a cramped examination room that the tech had led us to. I had a nervous smile twitching on my face as we waited, and waited, and waited. We were waiting too long and Christopher and I became restless when the doctor finally came in. Dr. Rox, who normally had a smile on his face and was always *'so happy to see you guys,'* had his face pulled into a tight, solemn grimace.

Ringing. Ringing. Ringing. My ears shrieked with the piercing sound of ringing. The air that I breathed in when I saw the look on the doctor's face when he walked into our tiny, stifling exam room had long since gone stale. I felt it stirring, welling, and building into a scream. Finally, it clawed out of my lungs in a sharp choke. Hot tears burned down my cheeks and dripped on my chest.

He said, "I'm so sorry. You need to prepare for the worst. Your baby will not make it."

There was nothing but ringing after that. Ringing and crying and a hole punched in my chest. I remember asking what exactly it was. He replied he just knew that the baby had measured small and there was something wrong with its spine and skull. There was a specialist in Wichita he went to school with who could tell us more. Then nothing more before he left the room. I felt the snipping of my worldly teacher being cut. I didn't reach for my husband but he came to me and held me while I sobbed.

A horrible whining sound escaped from my soul as I felt terror for my unborn baby. So many thoughts were racing my mind, *'This can't possibly be happening to us. We were out of the 13-week danger zone. What about Cayden who weeks earlier had been excited to be a big brother? How do we do this?'*

I could feel nothing but my heart breaking. I could feel cracks forming fissures in my being. We tried for our baby. We wanted our baby.

Minutes melted by. No one came to check on us, no comfort from the nurses or staff. It wasn't until Chris released me and said, "Let's go, we have to pick up Cayden."

That's when I stood up, my face swollen from tears, head wheeling, and knees weak. He took my hand. There was only one entrance and one exit at the clinic. This meant walking through the entire clinic to get to the car. I felt the pressure of his hand in mine and tried to focus on that but as my body moved through the clinic, it all passed in slow motion. The grave looks from the nurses, the whispers, pretending to look at charts but seeing me through the corner of their eyes. We almost made it to the first door when a nurse led a very pregnant woman through. Her glow was unmistakably dimmed when her eyes met mine filled with agony. Chris pulled me through the door to be met with the waiting room. The same weird smell burned my eyes now. But the sting could not numb the sensory overload that was a room full of happy expecting couples or a mother and her sweet newborn. I felt my punctured chest crack wide open. My essence flowed from it. The eyes, the silence, the pity filled my cavernous heart as it plunged into deeper despair.

Finally, we emerged from the double doors. The August Kansas sun blinded me in white. The heat stifled me and the humidity reminded me that I was still breathing and still pregnant. As we climbed into the car, Chris buckled my seatbelt. We left the parking lot and at Crawford Street, it felt like I came up for air after being held under the water. The ringing was muffled.

"I have to call Richard," I whispered to which Chris asked, "What?" "I have to call Richard, I am supposed to be at school today. I can't hold it together. I can't... see those kids."

I found Richard in my contacts and hit send. I hadn't thought about what I would say and that was my mistake in retrospect because when he answered with a, *"Hey Kelsey, what's up?"*

I promptly fell apart. I couldn't form words. I burst into tears all over again. *"Richard... my baby. There is something wrong with my baby."*

At that, he replied with the word of the day, *"What?"*

"We went to the doctor, there is something wrong with our baby. Richard, I can't go to that school."

"I'm so sorry Kelsey. I have it covered. Take care of yourself.

"Thank you," and I ended the call. It was all I could say.

Chris took me home. I was greeted by our two fluffy dogs and I climbed into bed fully clothed, pulled the covers over me, and felt my light go out. Chris asked what we should do about Cayden. I told him to call my dad and a few hours later he met him at the daycare. Chris explained to the childcare director what had happened and told her to remove our baby's place on the waitlist. I was grateful for his concern because if not, the call would've surely shattered me months later.

So there I laid in our bed, crying and telling myself to breathe.

Breathing and crying.

Crying and breathing.

Inside, the mother in me was screaming into an echo that could break the sky. She was strong and stood with defiance to her problems. While the storm raged, it tore her skirt and tattered her shirt, but she screamed. In the eyes of a tornado, at the bottom of the sea, she screamed. Fists raised at the lightning, eyes unblinking, she screamed.

Suddenly, the ground shifted and she stumbled. She was no longer screaming. She was suffocating as sand poured from her mouth, eyes burning, broken nails boring gashes into her lungs. Fighting but weakening as every breath went unanswered by the air… bleeding, reeling, and reaching for help.

And that was where I left her. The mother I was before we found out our baby would die. The happy—even when she struggled—mom. The mom that always made over-the-top birthday cakes. The working mom who wanted her babies to know everything the world has to offer. Who believed that to live was an adventure. She was who I abandoned at the bottom of the raging storm. That great tragedy roared in my subconscious as I laid inside our dark bedroom. On the outside, a single hot tear welled and fell from my right repent eye and onto my pillow.

It was one of the thousands, millions maybe that I cried not just for our baby but for the person I was before. The woman I would never see again. The mother who would return badly broken eventually. This was my process of "checking out." This was my untethering.

CHAPTER 2

We left for the hospital early that morning. We dropped Cayden off at the daycare and went on our way. It was an hour and a half drive and our appointment was at 9:00. I could tell Christopher was just as scared as I was. There wasn't a lot of talking. It had been a week since we received the terrifying report that our baby would not make it. We had been told that she was measuring small and there was something wrong with her spine as well as her skull. Those were our only precursors going into this day.

We begged the universe that the doctor was incorrect, he had some old equipment, and our baby would be okay. After all, they couldn't even see the baby's gender during that ultrasound. Maybe they didn't see our baby's anatomy correctly too.

We arrived at the hospital campus. It was huge for being in the middle of Kansas. We walked into the building, found the directory, and proceeded to the maternal-fetal specialist office. The building was old and made of brick and the carpet smelled musty in the elevator. Every step crept more anxiety and fear into my heart.

We were the first ones in the waiting room. We filled out some consent forms and obligatory paperwork but it wasn't long before we were called back by the ultrasound technician. She was cheery, which we later learned to be a facade. I used the bathroom before we started. The tech did not want me to pee on her chair, which was fair since it had been a long drive for a pregnant woman. When I came back, she had the room prepared. It was dark and felt huge compared to the ultrasound room in Salina. There was a large TV screen on the wall opposite to the chair and the ultrasound equipment so we would be able to see our baby on a large screen. Chris was seated next to the ultrasound chair. I laid back in the chair and pulled up my shirt, exposing my belly. A normal ultrasound, right? I wasn't prepared for how hard she pressed down onto my uterus. I knew that I had belly fat but she pressed the transponder hard against my abdomen. I felt the pressure bear down and it hurt.

The image of our baby soon popped up on the screen. We saw the profile of their face clearly. The ultrasound technician then walked us through the anatomy of our baby and took measurements. She showed us the heart first. Still beating and moving blood out to the body. Then she showed us their bladder, full of urine which meant they were practicing swallowing. I noticed though the farther and farther into the ultrasound we got, the quieter the technician got. She showed us the baby's hands and feet but it wasn't until we got to their arms and legs that we became alarmed. She remarked that she was measuring the baby's right ulna and we watched as she made three points at a 90-degree angle on the screen to measure. She measured the baby's tibia, once again making three points at a 90-degree angle. She measured the baby's femur and as she placed another set of three dots I asked, "You're measuring her whole leg, right?" To which she said that she wasn't. She was measuring the individual long bones. Horror and shock crossed my face. There was something very wrong with our baby. The technician asked if we wanted to know the gender to which we replied in affirmation. She told us, "It's a girl."

Chris held my hand to his cheek and sobbed. "Our little girl," he choked out, "Of course." Chris mourned his dream of having daddy's little girl. Something about knowing her gender made her a person. Made her more than just a baby—it was a part of us, and that part of us was very, very sick.

The ultrasound technician continued with the exam. "Her spine is not formed properly and her ribcage shows many breaks. Her body is a bell shape due to these breaks," she paused as she ran the transponder over her head.

She made a motion I could only describe as a 'bounce' against the side of my uterus and I saw our baby's skull flex. FLEX. Skulls don't flex. They are hard. More commentary from the ultrasound technician that, "The skull is flexible when probed with the transponder and is thin in formation." She bounced the transponder again and I cried out. There was no way it wasn't hurting our baby. It was her brain and her skull.

The technician finished her exam quietly and printed pictures of our baby for us. Tears painted our faces. Yes, something was wrong with our baby girl. We felt helpless and confused. She instructed us to return in two hours for our appointment with the doctor. *Two hours?'* I thought and then looked at the clock. It was already 12:00. That ultrasound had lasted three hours and my belly was sore from it. Though it could not compare to how sore my heart was after knowing something was wrong with our baby girl.

They told us to get lunch, I was still pregnant after all, and I must be hungry. We climbed into our Sorento. No, neither of us was hungry. We sat for a long time in the car before deciding on Jimmy John's and drove over. Chris was driving erratically, crying incoherently about our baby girl and I asked him to just turn around and go back to the parking lot. I wasn't hungry anyway and I was scared of him driving any further. When we waited in the parking lot we leaned the seats back in the car, expecting to get some rest when the phone rang. I looked at the clock. It had only been half an hour but it was the doctor's office asking us to come in.

We quickly left the car. Maybe there was nothing wrong and that's why they wanted us back so soon. Who was I kidding, though? We rode the lonely elevator up to the floor to an empty waiting room and were ushered straight back to a room. It was isolated at the end of a hallway. The room was clean enough, with floors that desperately needed wax. It had the standard gynecological exam table, chairs that I sat in, and a

TV screen with rotating images of medications, the hospital logo, and pregnant women. And so we waited.

⸺⊃∘⊂⸺

Christopher paced the room like a caged animal. They had called us far sooner than the two hours they had originally instructed. I cradled my belly—my baby girl instinctively. There was a knock on the door and Chris sat next to me. I wasn't prepared for what happened when the door opened.

The nurse entered first, white as a sheet, her smile now a tight grim line. Next came in a short plump woman with short burgundy hair. Her face was red because she was a redhead, right? The more I studied her in those seconds—that felt like hours—the more I realized that her face was not just red, it was puffy, and her makeup had a hint of tear wash to it. She had been crying and when we locked eyes I realized that she had been crying for me. The glassiness and the pain shown in her brown eyes were for me.

I rattled, pushed off my center. I was hoping that with the excitement of the baby being a girl may be there was a glimmer of hope that our baby would be okay. Maybe I needed extra help but it'd all be okay. That hope was crushed when I saw her eyes.

She identified herself as the doctor. She took my hands and I locked my eyes with hers. "There is no easy way to say this. Your baby has a rare genetic condition. She will not make it." My hands clutched hers as my whole world started to tip. She continued, "Your baby had Osteogenesis Imperfecta Type II, the lethal variant of brittle bone disease. As you saw in the ultrasounds, all of her long bones are broken into 90-degree angles, her ribs have broken several times already and had forced her body into a bell shape. I'm afraid it has caused her lungs to not develop and the ribs are crushing in on her heart. Her skull is deformed and is flexible around her brain. She won't survive gestation, if she is born, there is no record of life past 45 days."

I could feel black dots appearing in front of my vision that happens when I start to faint but I kept my eyes locked with hers. "What are our options?" Chris asked. "There are very few options. You can wait and see how far she progresses but her bones will continue to break as they form and she will pass away. Or you can terminate the pregnancy." "So an abortion?"

Chris asked. "Yes." "What do you recommend?" She returned her eyes to me.

"I would recommend terminating the pregnancy."

My ears were ringing again. "There's a chance that a broken bone of the baby could perforate your wife's uterus, causing internal bleeding." Her eye contact returned to my husband and he asked more questions. My hands cradled my belly. My baby. The ringing raged in my head as death was discussed around me. Images flashed in my head. All I wanted to do was claw my baby out of my skin and hold her safe in my arms. How could our baby be dying? Was it something I did? Not enough vitamins? I wanted her. We wanted her. How could we get an abortion? That was for women—other women—not me, right? We wanted her, tried for her, we got married months ago and we were doing things the 'right way.' Surely this wasn't true.

I wasn't aware of how much they had talked around me until the doctor patted my hand. "I'm so sorry, sweetheart," then she stood and left, the nurse following behind. I stared numb and terrified after them, tears silently flooding my cheeks. Christopher stood up and started pacing, a list of clinics that performed abortions in hand. I heard him call the first one and I hysterically fell apart. We had talked about this option before and confirmed it was what we would do if we had no other option. Well, we had no other option so he initiated the process to end our baby's suffering and save my life. He stared at me with fear in his eyes and ended the call. He told me he would be right back and left the room. I stared out the window, up at the sky, weeping and willing for that day to be a terrible dream. No such luck befell me. I felt the ground slip out from under me and my life falling apart.

Christopher came back in and relayed to me that it was going to be $2400 to go to Overland park or $1800 to go to Wichita. Either way, we couldn't afford it. They gave him a list of phone numbers for financial assistance for cases such as ours. I looked at the floor, defeated. We always made just marginally above the line for assistance, I wasn't prepared for rejection by people for this. I asked him if we could call them tomorrow, I just didn't have the strength for it the same day.

Chris agreed and took a seat next to me as we waited for the doctor to return. I was scared of the news she would bring back.

When she entered the room, she confirmed that we were going to take the only option we had and terminate the pregnancy. She recommended doing an amniocentesis to collect genetic data on the baby.

"It is a painless procedure," the doctor explained. "We insert a needle into your abdomen and extract some amniotic fluid from the uterus. This will give the genetic details we need to confirm the baby's diagnosis being a genetic condition." "Can't you just take a sample of her tissue after she passes? We don't want to put her through anything else," I asked. *Isn't breaking her bones by existing enough?'* I thought. The doctor gave me a look of pity, "Unfortunately, after the termination, there is no guarantee that the doctor will collect a tissue sample. The only guarantee is to get a genetic sample now, while she is still in-utero." My eyes pricked with tears as she continued, "You should know there is a chance that the amniocentesis will cause preterm labor. Especially in cases where the pregnancy is unstable." I felt my eyes widen, we could meet our baby today, and this could be over today. Not over but the fear and sorrow for our baby's suffering would come to an end.

"With everything I just told you, do you still want to go through with the amniocentesis?" she asked.

I looked at my husband's face, he too was holding back tears. "Yes, we need to know so we will do the amniocentesis." "Good, I have a couple of patients I need to do before we do the test. In the meantime, we will have you speak to the geneticist so that you can learn more about your baby's condition. You can head over now. They are expecting you."

"Okay," Chris said. We rose from our chairs we had felt implanted in while she gave Chris directions to the geneticist's office. It was across the street in a separate building that we could reach through the tunnel.

We were led through a back hallway to the exit. In hindsight, I was thankful I wouldn't have to see more pregnant women. As we walked in silence the tears streamed down my face. Why us? Why our baby? This was the stuff of horror films except no film or book has dared to touch this disease.

When we arrived at the geneticist we were not prepared for the waiting room. It was a pediatric geneticist. The room was filled with toys while small patients were busy playing with them. Those were children living with genetic disorders. Just a glimmer of hope that the doctor got it wrong. That our baby could survive despite the genetic anomaly. We told the receptionist our names and they apologized for us having to see the other patients and immediately ushered us into a room far at the end of the hallway. No, this was most certainly not good news.

I looked at my phone. It was already 2:00. I texted my dad that we still had two more appointments. I asked him if he could pick up Cayden from daycare and we would just pick him up from their house the next day. He replied that he would. I looked up. More white walls met my gaze. Chris was on his phone doing something so I sat in silence until the doctor came in, which wasn't that long. No, you never want to be the top priority on a doctor's list. It means you are really, truly fucked.

The doctor came in with a grave look on her face. When you break not one or two health professional's poker faces but four you are fucked. I learned that from my brother George's lifelong battle being born with only one ventricle.

The doctor sat on a chair and shared that she had received the ultrasound images and confirmed our maternal-fetal doctor's diagnosis. She reiterated that the baby was most likely not survive through the in-utero or, if born, she would suffocate from undeveloped lungs, trapped by her continually breaking ribcage, shortly after birth. Her case was severe so she was confident that she would pass away in-utero at any time. A pain stung in my chest as she continued to tell us the mechanisms of the disease of which I had to look up later because I couldn't comprehend what she was saying past the news about our baby. She said that it was not our fault that this happened. She assured us that it was a random genetic anomaly. It happens to one in two million babies. It is not something that we carry with us because of the fetal fatality nature of the condition but now that we have a baby with the condition there was a slight increase in the possibility of having another baby with the condition.

I honestly don't remember much after that part of the conversation. I felt lost. There was no one to blame, not even ourselves to blame for the position our baby was in. It was just a random thing… then why us? Why our baby?

The geneticist assured us that they would analyze the sample from the amniocentesis and asked to take my blood as well for further genetic analysis. We agreed and were escorted through a back hallway to the exit. We needed to get back across the street for the amniocentesis. We walked in silence. Tears falling quietly. Inside the waiting room for the maternal-fetal doctor, we went where we were met with more pregnant women. The receptionist ushered us back right away, I heard her apologize to the patients in the waiting room for me. I must have scared them. I was scared of myself.

They took us back to the ultrasound room we had started our day in. We would get to see our baby one more time. They laid me flat on the chair that had been converted into a bed. The ultrasound tech was preparing instruments I had not noticed before. The doctor came in with several sterile packages and a preloaded syringe. The doctor came up to my head and placed her hand on my shoulder. "Now the anesthetic may sting and you may feel a pinch of the needle going in but this should not hurt. There is a chance it may hurt but I have done this for a very long time, and I have never had a patient hurt," she said with a tender look on her face. I could feel her sympathy for me radiate off of her. "Are you ready?" she asked. "Are you sure this won't hurt the baby?" I questioned back. "No, it won't hurt the baby. Are you ready?" "No, but let's get this done." Then she pulled out the needle. The big fucking needle. This needle was thick enough you could stick pencil lead into it.

I squirmed in my skin. She put it on the tray and picked up the iodine. She had me pull up my shirt and wiggle my pants down over my hips to expose my belly. She draped a blue paper cloth over me, leaving the procedure field exposed and she rubbed it down thoroughly with iodine to prevent infection since the needle would be going into my body past my skin. She then picked up the pre-loaded syringe that she identified as the anesthetic and administered it. Yes, there was a pinch and a fiery burn that marginally spread. She waited a few minutes to let it "do its job."

The ultrasound technician picked up the gloved transponder and held it to my belly, opposite from the injection. There was our baby on the big screen again. Knowing what I knew about how much pain she was in, made tears fall from my eyes again. "I am going to insert the amnio needle now, this shouldn't take long," she reassured.

Chris held my hand and I watched her bring the needle to my skin. I then turned my gaze to the ceiling, trying to picture my peaceful memory. That's when I felt the needle pierce my skin. I looked into Chris' eyes in a panic. The needle burned as it went in. I felt it struggle through my fat layer and get stuck on my abdominal muscles. I was being stabbed. Actually fucking stabbed and I had never felt this kind of pain before. Not with my pain injections. Not with the car accident I was in. Not even with my labor with Cayden. I felt her push the needle in harder and my muscles to make way for the needle. I then felt the resistance of the needle on my uterus. I thought I was going to vomit; I was sobbing from the pain. Finally, she pushed the needle through my uterus. She kept saying, "I've never had anyone hurt before, I am so sorry, honey." All I could feel was the burning of the needle in my belly. She tried to tell me that the pain in my heart was so much worse than the pain of the needle. I told her that it was pretty damn close. I didn't move my body but my toes curled from the pain and I gripped Chris' hand like a lifeline.

They took the fluid from my uterus and removed the needle slowly. I could feel the relief of my uterus and my muscles relaxing and rolled my head back and forth when the needle was finally out, and they were applying pressure to the site.

The doctor squeezed my shoulder softly, "I am so sorry, sweetheart. It is over now. I am so sorry I hurt you. Make sure you rest now." "Except now I get to go do a blood draw. More needles. Yay," I spat sarcasm through my tears. They wiped down my belly and pulled my shirt back down. It hurt to sit up and it felt like my guts were wrenching when I turned my body to swing my legs over the side of the table. The procedure was over though. We would get answers about our baby but not for several months. The ultrasound technician gave us directions to the lab and ushered us out through the back door so we wouldn't have to face the lobby again.

I was still crying, overwhelmed by the day. The diagnosis of our baby, the pain of the amniocentesis, the fracturing of my heart with every step that day. When the lab technician saw me she tried to make a joke to lighten the mood. "Now I haven't even stuck you, so you can't cry yet," she said with a bright tone. "We just got done with an amniocentesis," Christopher growled. "Oh," the tech replied, "Those are no fun. I'm sorry that I have to stick you again." She was quiet then. She pulled out several tubes and one butterfly needle. She pressed it into my vein. Just a pinch, my body was still in pain and reeling from the procedure before so it did not hurt. She wished us a better day and we left.

We walked out of the building, it was past 5:00. Our day of torture was over but the pain in our hearts was just getting started. We climbed into the car in silence. I whimpered from the overwhelming day and sobbed. It wasn't enough that our baby was going to die, but she was suffering so much. We were going to have to terminate the pregnancy or risk my life too. How could we do that?

I don't remember if it was Christopher or I who texted my dad to tell him about the diagnosis and what our only option was. All I remember is that he got the message. He had picked up Cayden and brought him home as promised so we would not have to face our son after that long day.

We were on the highway back home when Chris took my hand, tears falling down his cheeks. "Can we name her Hope?"

he asked through the pain in his heart, "I just think her name should be Hope. She was our Hope for the future." "Of course," I sobbed, "Can her middle name be Charlotte? I've always wanted a little I could call Charlie." "Yes, we can," He kissed my hand that he was holding. We held onto each other's hands for dear life during that car ride.

I texted my boss Wendy to let her know that we were going to lose our little girl and asked for more time off, to which she obliged. I was relieved by the mercy, but conscious of the fact that I did not have any paid time off banked yet. I didn't know how to face my job, though—so many children, and so many adults that looked to me for answers. All I could focus on was the next horrific thing.

We had to terminate our pregnancy.

We took our time getting up the next morning. Our son, Cayden, would be swimming and eating ice cream at his grandparent's house and probably didn't want to be disturbed. We drove the hour to Manhattan, Kansas, where my parent's house was located.

My chest sunk at the thought of getting out of the car. We had texted the diagnosis to my parents the night before and if they did what we did—Googled it—they would have been horrified by the images related to Osteogenesis Imperfecta Type II. We would have to talk to my parents about the disease, about our only option. We would need financial help. A termination was $1,800 in Wichita and $2,400 in Overland Park. Any way you put it, we couldn't afford it. We were given a list of places that could give us a scholarship. So, that day was spent calling those places. Time was not on our side as 20th week was approaching quickly.

We walked up the hill to my parents' house and let ourselves in. As we thought, they were in the pool. We sat outside and watched them for a little while before my mom excused herself, telling my dad that he was in charge of Cayden and invited us to talk inside. She went to change and we sat on her couch. 'Couch' seemed too underwhelming of a term for the piece we were sitting on. It was a monstrosity of a sectional that took up most of the room, always had disheveled pillows and a long tear on the back from a once notorious pug long since passed. Damn, I missed that pug.

My mom came out and sat across from us in a chair. "Well Kelsey, it just sucks," she started. "It is just horrible and I am so sorry for you and for you Chris. Your Dad and I looked up the disease last night and the chance of survival was zero. That is just terrible." "I know, mom, there is nothing we can do to help her," I interrupted. "Your dad and I talked about it and we will pay for the abortion." Shock crept on my face as that was something I would have never expected, and she continued, "We see it as saving your life because we can't save your baby's life. Something really terrible could happen to you if you try to carry this baby and we just don't want that to happen and we know you don't have the money so we will pay for it." I got up and hugged my mother around the neck and sobbed. "We are doing it because we love you, Kelsey. We don't want anything bad happening to you. We can't save your baby but we can save you. Never had I ever thought that I would pay for an abortion. I don't believe in it. I'm a devout Catholic, you know. But I don't see it that way... I see it as saving your life and sometimes you have to do what you have to do to save your life. We can't save your baby. I'm sorry, Kelsey."

For the first time in a long time, it really felt like my mom really, truly cared about me and my well-being. More than just on her terms but as a daughter. "We are still trying to get the financial assistance so maybe it won't come to that," I said through the tears. She replied, "You can try but we will do it either way. I will also book you a hotel room so you won't have to travel the same day. I want you to go to Overland Park. I already looked it up. If anything bad happens to you, you stand a better chance in Kansas City than in Wichita, Kansas. Please go to Overland Park." "We will," Chris and I reassured her. "Thank you, this means so much to us."

Chris and I went into my Mom's office on the same floor and called the financial aid places. Even though I made a pretty meager wage working for a nonprofit, it was still enough for one counselor to laugh at me when I asked for financial aid. Every single call went either unanswered or rejected or it would take too long to get a response. The last call we made was to the Overland Park Clinic. "I can get you in on Friday," the voice said. To which I asked, "This Friday?" "Yes, this Friday. You will need to bring the full payment with you and we would recommend paying for the follow-up appointment in advance as well. You will also have the option to cremate the pregnancy tissue, would you want to do that?" My brain went numb at that phrase being used for our baby. Nonetheless, I responded, "Yes, we want her cremated and her ashes back." "Please bring the full payment, and do not eat after 8:00 PM the night before. We will see you at 7:30 AM this Friday morning." "Thank you," I got in before the line went dead.

We went out and told my mom, she immediately booted up her slow computer and booked a hotel room for us for Thursday and Friday night. We were thankful for that. They said they would take Cayden, so we just had to drop him off on

——————∞——————

our way to Overland Park.

I felt broken as we waited for Friday. I was barely hanging onto my sanity, moving through motions. I clung to the family that we did have. I held Cayden extra tight for every hug and snuggled extra on the couch for our evening TV time. During the day, Chris looked at me with pain in his eyes, like I was a ticking time bomb. At night, he held me until he fell asleep, I knew he still cared. Before he came home from work and when Cayden fell asleep, the fluffy dogs piled on top of my legs and laid next to me on the couch.

On Tuesday night, I researched urns for our baby's ashes. Did you know that most people don't cremate when an infant dies? There is a chance you may get no ashes back because the bones are so soft still. It was a risk that we were taking to possibly not get any of Hope's ashes but I could not stand the thought of burying her somewhere and not being able to visit her or see her grave while I was mourning. I just couldn't leave her somewhere when my job required us to move every three years.

When it came to the urns they were hundreds or thousands of dollars. We could never afford one, and I didn't want to ask our family for one more thing. GoFundMe occurred to me but I couldn't stand not telling Hope's full story when asking for other people's money. Most were adult sizes which seemed so big for our little baby. They were also dark and garish looking, so heavy for our little sweet baby. Our baby deserved better.

During my research, I found that some mothers put their baby's ashes in ornate jewelry boxes or keepsake boxes because they too felt that urns were too dark for the memorial of their angel babies. Being in the middle of Kansas, our retail opportunities were limited. I pulled up Amazon and typed in "ornate jewelry boxes." A variety popped up on the screen but a small, beautiful silver-plated one with a red velvet lining stood out. There was even space for us to engrave her name on the top. It was an option we could afford so I ordered it. A hot tear fell down my cheek and I touched my belly.

"It just isn't fucking fair," I whispered. I should be planning a gender reveal for her, not her funeral arrangements. "I am so sorry, Hope." I felt her moving and kicking less and less during those days. It made sense, every movement hurt her and her bones broke more and more every day. My poor sweet baby.

I didn't know that funeral arrangements would be this hard. I think the problem was my honesty. I was honest about why I needed my baby's ashes blessed and why I couldn't have the body before for that. I had told them that I had to terminate our pregnancy due to a fatal genetic condition that was breaking our baby's bones and that she had been suffering. I know, I know... don't talk to Christians about terminating a pregnancy but I wanted to be honest. I didn't want to lie to God's messengers to get her ashes blessed or prayed over. There also was no Jewish establishment in Salina, Kansas, or I would have just gone straight there.

The first church I called was nondenominational. The phone rang and an older woman answered; I told her that I was losing my baby and that I needed to talk to the pastor. She put me right through. He listened to my whole story before replying flatly that they simply don't bless ashes or pray for aborted babies there before hanging up the phone.

I called six more churches... avoiding the Catholic and Southern Baptist ones. However, they were all the same. A few even told me that I was going to hell and so was my baby. That even included some of the pastors I knew through the partnerships at my job—the ones I considered good people and friends. I guess when it really came down to it, I was in the middle conservative Bible belt and there were no loving hands of God to bless my baby for a safe journey to the afterlife.

No matter how hard I tried, there would be no funeral for our baby to memorialize her short, painful life and that hurt me. My mom once told me that you don't go to the funeral just for the dead, but also for the living who need love and support. I wanted people to know that Hope's life mattered and I needed the love from our village to help me get through that painful time.

I never got that chance. No church would accept my plea and funeral homes were far, far past our price point. I think that's why writing this book is so important to me. This is my eulogy for my sweet baby, Hope. It's my cry as a mother to tell the world that my baby mattered and what happened to us was unjust.

CHAPTER 3

I don't remember falling asleep the previous night but I do remember waking up early that morning. I pulled my toiletries from the suitcase and climbed into the shower. As I felt the water wash down my body, the numbness in my surroundings started creeping into my soul until it had completely encapsulated my entire existence. A hard ringing buzzed in my ears. That was it. That was the day our baby was about to die. As the reality settled into my consciousness, I instinctively stopped breathing. I had noticed that I could rarely feel her move lately. I couldn't blame her. Every movement could break a bone, every breath cracked a rib, and every head bobble was compression on her brain.

"All she knows is pain," I whispered to myself.

I loved the little baby inside me but I knew that the only way I could give her relief was by letting her go.

The water cascaded from the shower down my face and mingled with the unstoppable hot tears that kept on escaping my eyes.. Fear set in. My grandmother had died years earlier from a surgical procedure gone wrong. I had my own scare with my C-section from the time I had Cayden. Surgery in itself was terrifying… but surgery outside of a hospital where there are no lifesaving instruments seemed much worse.

My fear for my baby was very real. I knew that we had to terminate the pregnancy to end her suffering and to save my life… but at what cost? What exactly was the procedure? I didn't know. Even when I tried to research, propaganda and disturbing images littered the internet. What was real? What was not? Dilation and curettage was for earlier pregnancies. Dilation and evacuation was what I would be put through later that day. What did it even mean, though? Maybe it was best I didn't know but the fear of the unknown gave me crippling anxiety.

I turned off the water and stepped out of the shower, dried off, and put on some foundation. I didn't put on regular makeup. It didn't make sense to do so. I let my black hair down from the top knot on my head. I put on loose black yoga pants and a black t-shirt. I knew I wanted to be as comfortable as possible for that day in hell. When I checked my phone, I saw that my mother had left messages for me and a text to let me know that my dad had left early in the morning and would meet us at the clinic. All I had to do was to text him the address. They wanted to make sure we weren't harassed by protesters and my father was a giant man who can fill up a doorway. Between him and my six-foot-five husband, people should leave us alone. That and a part of me just wanted my daddy in the face of that new fear.

While I was checking my phone, Christopher took his turn in the shower and got dressed. We barely talked as we were already agitated about what lies ahead. We went to the car and made our way to the clinic. I didn't see my Dad's jeep in the parking lot but I also did not see any protesters yet. *"I guess 7:30 AM is too early for them,"* I flippantly thought but was thankful for not having to face a bunch of psychopaths.

We walked inside and upon identifying myself to the receptionist, we were ushered into another room situated within the waiting room. The room was secluded as it had a door that locked behind the waiting room, and there were no windows so we had complete privacy. I began crying fearing what might happen next. An administrator came in. She was an older lady with white curly hair. "Oh sweetheart, I'm sorry. I understand you are here for a dilation and evacuation today, is that correct," she placed her hand on my knee and spoke in a kind tone, "Tell me what brought you here." I explained Hope's genetic condition and how much pain she was in. I explained how my parents were helping financially with the procedure because we did not qualify for financial aid even though I worked for a nonprofit and my husband worked as a janitor for an elementary school. "You may not have qualified over the phone but after talking to you now, I think we can help. We have people who donate to the clinic to help people like you who are in a hard position. Would $800 help you to be able to pay for it?" I cried harder and between sobs said, "Yes, that would make a huge difference. Thank you so much."

At that moment, there was a knock at the door. The nurse opened the door to be met by my Dad who -as usual- filled up the door way. The look of sadness when his eyes met mine was hardly bearable. I identified him as my dad and told the nurse that he could come in. The already small room felt cramped with the four of us inside it. The administrator continued, "So, we recommend prepaying for your follow up appointment after the procedure. Would you like to do that?" "Yes, we will do that," my dad chimed in. Christopher had been completely silent for most of the conversation which confused me. He was completely zoned out, I guess that was his way of helping himself, by checking out. I wish I had that luxury

I answered some more questions and then took my Mom's credit card from the folder she had prepared for us. The administrator left to run the card for over $1400. I sobbed and my Dad lightly rubbed his hand on my back. A nurse came in next, asking for a urine sample to run a urinalysis. They needed to make sure I was not under the influence of drugs or alcohol. I was deeply insulted but understood that they had a significant amount of hoops they had to jump through to stay open. I guess making sure that those asking for a termination are sober is one of those hoops. I went into the bathroom that was just one door over to give my sample. Zika Virus and your pregnancy posters covered the bathroom walls and stall door.

When I returned, the administrator had come back in with a card. She asked me to write a "thank you" to the donors that had provided the funding to help pay for my procedure. My tears were hot in my eyes as I wrote, *"Thank you for your donation. It means so much to our family..."* and something along the lines of thank you for your help. Our baby was suffering. *Was suffering.* Past tense. She was still suffering now and would for a few more hours. The administrator told us to wait in the small room and then we would be called back to the exam room.

My Dad stayed out in the waiting room when we were called back. I was guessing that he just felt claustrophobic. I later found out from my Mom that he had stepped out to call her. He was crying himself and wanted to remain strong for me.

The nurse weighed me and took my vitals. She led us back to another tiny room. That was for the ultrasound. She instructed me to remove my pants and cover myself with a paper cloth. Chris helped me take my pants off and climb up onto the table. We waited until a doctor entered the room. She was in her 50s, kept her hair in a tight bun, and was dressed in scrubs with a white lab coat on top. She honestly reminded me of my aunt with her mannerism. She introduced herself and said, "Today is going to be a horrible day. There is just no way around it. We will try to make it less horrible but overall... It will just be a horrible day. If you accept it, it will get just a little easier." I was crying and gurgled out an "okay." The doctor looked concerned and asked, "Are you sure you want to do this?" To which I responded, "Yes, I want to end our baby's suffering. I am just really sad." "Now under state law I am required to do an ultrasound to confirm gestational age. Would you like to see the screen while I do it? Keep in mind this is a much, much older machine than the one in Wichita. I received your ultrasound images from them. I am so sorry about what has happened. Do you want to see the ultrasound?" I replied, "No." I was too much of a coward to face the broken bones again and our baby's suffering. She told me she understood and ran the transponder over my belly.

"Wow, this is what Osteogenesis Imperfecta Type II looks like. I have only ever read about it in textbooks. It is so rare. Yes, it looks like you are a little over 18 weeks according to this ultrasound." She pulled the transponder away and printed the images before attaching them with a paperclip to my file. She wiped off my belly and helped me sit up. "Now, I will tell you what the procedure will be like. We will start by inserting a speculum. We will then add anesthetic to your cervix. Then, I'm going to insert several bamboo rods into your cervix to break your water. This will help dilate your cervix so we can get the baby out. After that, you will go back to where you are staying for a few hours while your cervix dilates. When you come back, we will remove the bamboo shoots and check on your dilation. It is normal to feel cramps or contractions because we are basically inducing labor. We will then remove all of the pregnancy tissues and eliminate what needs to be suctioned to prevent infection. You will not be completely unconscious for this but we will give you medication to help you forget and relax, and give you painkillers for some relief. Do you have any questions?"

I paused while my brain spun with the information, "Will Chris be able to be there with me?" I asked because Chris had once again been absent in the conversation. "For the first part he will be allowed back there but for the second part, he will not. While we will give you medication to help you forget, we are not able to give him the same medication. He would remember everything and that isn't fair. So, for the second part he will wait in the waiting room." My heart dropped and my spine prickled with fear.

"What about the baby? Will I be able to see her after," I asked. To which she replied with a very flat 'no.' She told me that there was no guarantee what condition the body would be in and it could cause me more harm than good to see her. They were going to provide us with a couple of keepsakes afterwards to memorialize our baby but I would not be able to see her. My stomach twisted in knots. No guarantee on what condition the body would be in. I felt like throwing up but instead I just cried more.

"Are you sure that you want to go through with it?" the doctor asked again. I wish she would fucking stop asking. "Yes, I am sure," I responded through my tears. "Okay, I will write you a prescription for antidepressants and antibiotics. Do not hesitate and start taking these right away. It will help you cope with the next several months and the antibiotics will help kill any infection that can arise. Take the medication. Do not wait," she urged. "I will also give you a sheet with phone numbers. One is a psychiatrist here in Overland Park. I recommend especially for you to seek out therapy right away since you have a history of depression and anxiety. The other phone numbers are the abortive support and suicide hotline, and our phone number. Please call only these numbers and if you find yourself in an emergency after the procedure call us and come see us. Do not go to the ER. They will not understand the procedure you just went through and can make it worse if they are not educated."

"Call only you guys for emergencies, call only the people on this list for help. Okay, I got it," I responded. "And take the medication." "And take the medication," I replied. I could afford the antibiotic but the antidepressant would have to wait until my next paycheck. The doctor told us she was going to check on the room and the staff and she would be back when they were ready for us.

Chris helped me put my pants back on to walk down the hallway but we weren't saying much to each other. I felt that the foundation of our relationship had started to shake. We were turning away from each other instead of turning towards each other. The nurse came in to get us and led us down the hall. Every step felt like it was longer than the last, the hallway was beginning to turn on end and all I could hear was my heavy breath. At last, we arrived at the last room at the very end of the hallway. The room was even smaller than the previous one.

A nurse brought in some paperwork for us to fill out. It expressed written consent for the procedure. *"Pretty standard,"* I thought. I was caught off guard by the next page though. It was the funeral home order form. I had to check that we wanted Hope's remains cremated, not buried. I had to check that I wanted her remains cremated by herself and that I wanted the ashes back. I had to sign a release saying that because she was so small and underdeveloped we may not get any ashes back. I said a prayer before signing that line. I also had to sign that the cremation fee of $260 needed to be paid before cremation would be performed. I signed it, hoping that my dad or someone would be able to help us with this expense. Next, we had to write in her name. I wrote in 'Hope' and broke down in incoherent tears. I couldn't remember how to spell Charlotte. I spelled and misspelled and crossed it out and rewrote it maybe five times. I was so overwhelmed. Finally, I filled out both Christopher and my names and date of births and signed the form. I handed the clipboard back to the nurse who lightly squeezed my shoulder.

Once again, I was instructed to remove my pants and cover with a paper sheet. I did as I was instructed, weeping every step of the way. This was it. This would be the end of our journey with baby Hope. Her suffering would come to an end and ours would just be beginning. The doctor came in with three staff members this time. One was a resident doing her rotation and the other two were nurses. The room felt like the worst version of a clown car and I was the main event.. Of all the times to decide you are a teaching clinic, now? On the worst goddamn day of my life? I didn't have time to argue. The doctor instructed me to move my backside down so that my bottom was at the edge of the table. She told me she would relay everything she was doing so I did not have any surprises.

She then inserted a cold, metal speculum inside me and cranked it open. Uncomfortable as hell but I was hanging in. Then I caught sight of the anesthetic needle. Another giant needle. She then inserted that needle into my cervix. "Fuck," I gasped, "Fuck, fuck, fuck!" Chris stood up from his chair to hold my hand. In the other hand, I held my grandmother's locket tightly. I felt a burning sensation inside me as if a small sharp fire was lit there. They paused to let the anesthetic spread.

The doctor looked at me, "Okay, for the last time, this is it. Are you sure you want to go through with this?" "Yes," I choked out through a sob, "I don't want her to hurt anymore!" She inserted a small hook and broke my waters. I felt a small gush and then pressure as she inserted bamboo shoots into the opening. I could feel every single one getting irreverently shoved in there to open my cervix up. While it didn't hurt per say, every single one made me want to crawl out of my skin as I felt it wrench my cervix open. She inserted a dozen shoots into a hole that was barely the size of a pencil tip when she began. She was finally done with part one.

We needed to wait three hours before coming back to complete the procedure. It was important we were back on time because the small pain medication they gave me would wear off and the bamboo shoots needed to be removed in precisely three hours to work the best they could, and to also prevent infection. I agreed as the doctor and nurse helped me sit up. I felt very strange. Nauseous but also a stiffness in my lower abdomen. When they helped me stand my legs shook uncontrollably. They said it was most likely due to the anesthetic but it would wear off. They led us out the back door of the hallway to the far-side of the waiting room where my Dad was anxiously waiting. Chris debriefed him that it wasn't over, that we needed to come back in three hours to complete the procedure. My Dad agreed to follow us over to the hotel and wait with us.

I got into our car with difficulty. My legs were still shaking and my stiff abdomen made getting into the car especially difficult. Chris drove over to the hotel that was one exit away from the clinic. He didn't say anything. I yelped multiple times at every single bump on the road as it felt like the shoots were shifting.

When we finally arrived at the hotel, my dad was standing there holding his laptop bag and we led up to our room. It was noon and I knew Chris and my dad would be hungry. I was worried about Chris eating because I needed him to stay awake and focused for me. I also really wanted some time alone to relax without having to worry about him and just worry about myself. So, I pressed my dad to take Chris somewhere to eat.

My dad practically dragged Chris out of the hotel room. Chris' concern was understandable but my Dad heard my message loud and clear. I needed a few moments alone with my baby. Was I selfish? Maybe. But at that moment, I needed to take care of myself and feel the way I wanted to feel without apologizing or comforting anyone else. I inhaled and exhaled a deep sigh.

I slipped off my shoes and felt the carpet beneath my swollen feet. I quietly padded over to the leather armchair. I pulled it over to the window so I could see the sky. The tears came rushing once more as I held my belly, Hope's feet drummed lightly in response. I let myself loose to beg, pray, and feel what I needed. I was in the fox hole, the bombs were dropping so I surrendered myself to God and my family that had already passed.

First I begged God, "Please, please take my baby Hope into heaven. Let her feel no more pain. She is so wanted and so loved. Please, please God take my baby so she can be at peace. Take her and do what you want with me. Take her where she is safe and can no longer get hurt."

I was sobbing now at my pitiful plea to a God whose existence I grappled with just weeks earlier. Would he listen to me? Would he lovingly take my baby into his kingdom? I had to believe so because I could feel my mind and soul shredding to pieces as my actions tried to find their space in my mind.

My tears were pooling on my chest, falling in steady streams from my eyes. I turned my attention to my relatives that had already passed on.

"Grandma, if you are listening out there, I need you to hear me now," I pleaded to the sky. "I couldn't let Hope suffer anymore, Grandma. I had to let her go. Please take her into your arms, Grams. Please love her with everything you have. Please hold her and tell her that her mother, father, and brother love her. Please, please find a place in your heart for her and hold her close until we can see her again. Have her meet Grandma Adelle and have her feed her French fries and listen to the polka. Spoil her like you spoiled me with Grandma Winnie and Aunt Dorothy," I begged, "Above all, please love her. Love her the way you loved me, only more. Treat her like a doll and dress her in the fashions you always wanted. Teach her to ride, cook, and run and have her feel no pain. Just please hold her and love her."

At last, I gazed down at my burgeoning belly underneath my fingertips. Hope's kicks were fading slowly. That is when I addressed her and said, "Hi baby. I am so… so sorry…" my voice cracked as my heart broke open and I cried harder than I ever had in my entire life. "Now, you be good for your Grandmas and your aunts, and oh, Tigger. Don't forget to play with him, he will bring you so many laughs. I wish I could keep you but you are hurting so much, sweetheart. It would be selfish for me to keep you here. I love you so much. Your daddy loves you and so does your big brother. I'm so sorry. I'm sorry," I cried as I felt her gentle thumps that had started become slower until I couldn't feel them anymore. I knew she was gone then. I cradled my belly and sobbed. "I love you," I whispered through my tears. I rocked back and forth as sobs racked my body over and over grieving until they came to a solemn end.

I felt cramps building up, like horrible period cramps at first. My abdomen and my cervix started hurting so I climbed into bed and tried not to move. Only an hour had passed before Chris flung open the door and climbed in bed next to me. My Dad remained in the lobby, to get some work done. Part of me wondered if he was ashamed of me but also wondered how he could just be working today.

Three hours. They said come back in three hours. I looked at the clock and meditated. Chris sat by my side in bed. He turned on the Harry Potter marathon to have something on. I withdrew from the world and focused on my breath.

The problem with Harry Potter is that it gets vibrant and loud during the action scenes. With every "expelliarmus" and basilisk, I broke my breath. The images of Harry Potter becoming interlaced with my pain and the loss of Hope. I tried with my whole mind to focus on my breath. Just like my labor with Cayden. When a wave of pain rushed through my body from head to toes, I closed my eyes and turned inward. With each inhale, I breathed in the pain, embracing it. I pictured my memory and breathed the pain out.

What was the memory I clung to, you may ask? When I was 19, I worked at the crown jewel of outdoor experiences. 221 square miles of land in Northern New Mexico. We hiked to the top of a mountain in just three hours that day. My very first mountain. We ate lunch, sang a Michelle Branch song. My heart was buzzing with happiness and warmth. We laid on the rocks that day, looking at a perfect blue sky. The sun kissed my face, the breeze tickled the hair across my cheek, and the boulders felt cool on my back. That moment of peace is frozen forever in my memory ever since.

I used this memory in biofeedback sessions, to try to lessen my existing chronic pain with some success. It was this memory I turned to during my pain injections, my labor with Cayden, and it was the memory I turned to now.

Meditating helped the time go by quicker. At 2:45, my cramps had developed into full blown contractions. My belly squeezed into a hard ball at regular intervals by then. It was time to get back to the clinic. My Dad drove Christopher and me because he didn't believe either of us should be driving. I got into the back of the car with much work. My contractions were getting harder and worse. I cried out in agony when my dad hit pot holes. My dad apologized profusely. I just wanted to crawl out of my own skin. I was losing control.

When we arrived at the clinic, Chris and my dad helped me out of the jeep, standing on both sides, taking hold of each arm, and leading me towards the front door. The receptionist looked scared and led us to the first room we waited in, secluded from the waiting room. I had to pee so I walked myself over to the bathroom that was just one door over. I went, reading the Zika Virus literature again. My pee was dark yellow because I had not eaten or drank anything in close to 18 hours.

I guess we were in the wrong room because when I returned to our waiting room, a nurse showed up to take us back. We went back to the same tiny room where we had been about three hours earlier. They instructed me once again to take off my pants. My dad waited outside the door as Chris helped me with my pants. They also told me to remove all my jewelry, in the event that I had to receive emergency assistance AKA an AED, it would burn me if I had jewelry present. I reluctantly took off my locket and strung my wedding bands on the chain before handing them to Christopher. I sat with another paper cloth over my legs and my Dad came back in. I was already crying again, from fear and the excruciating pain. He rubbed my back and Christopher held my hand. The nurse came back in and reported that the doctor was tied up in an emergency at that moment so I would have to wait a little bit, but there was no sense in me suffering anymore. I could have the medication that would help me relax, make me sleepy, and help me forget the procedure all together.

Dehydration 101. Blood vessels sink into your body when you are dehydrated to try to conserve fluids. Someone should have taught this nurse this simple concept before she attempted to place my IV. She blew one vein in my arm, a second in my other arm. My Dad spoke up, "Don't you think you should use a butterfly since she is so dehydrated?" to which the nurse replied that she had the medical degree while she blew the vein in my hand up. She then left the room and returned with the butterfly that she finally placed on my right hand. I could tell she was perturbed that my Dad had been correct. She hooked the IV bag to my port and I felt a rush of cold as the saline and medication entered my veins. I started shivering and shaking uncontrollably. She told us that it was a very normal reaction to the medication and assured us that she would get me a blanket before leaving the room, promising to be back very soon.

I was shaking but I tried to force a smile for Chris and my Dad who stared back at me with concern. I was still in labor but the medicine was making me less anxious about it and took the edge off of the pain. Dad grumbled about the dumbass nurse as we waited for her to return

We waited for almost an hour.

Christopher and Dad were getting more and more anxious as I started to soar sky high from the medication but still paused, writhed, and breathed through contraction pain. I don't remember who went to get the nurse, my dad or Chris, but one of them left the room to track her down. I was waiting too long for what was supposed to be a time-sensitive procedure. They came back in with the nurse.

She apologized for the delay, explaining that there was a medical emergency the doctor and staff had been tied up in. Wouldn't I want the doctor to take her time with me if that was the case? Dad said, "That's fine but we could've used an update. Also, where was the blanket you told you were going to get?"

I was still shaking from the medication.

She left and quickly came back with a plush red blanket. I told her that now I really had to pee since I had been waiting for so long. She said she wasn't sure that was possible since I was hooked up to the IV and to heart monitor leads. I was so out of it that I hadn't even noticed they had placed leads on me. The nurse left again.

She returned with help. First, they could not let me wander the halls without pants on. They wrapped the plush red blanket around my waist. Next, they disconnected my heart leads and took down my IV bag. One nurse held my leads and bag and the other locked arms with me. I was still contracting so I needed help to walk. The one with the IV bag popped her head out of the door, when she deemed the coast was clear they led me down a part of the hallway that I had not been in yet. I don't think anyone had been in yet actually. I could tell it was under construction by the nurse sweeping back the plastic tarp and the fact that there was no floor, just bare cement. I was also barefoot so the cool concrete felt nice.

I had them pause walking as a large contraction waved through my body. I mean my whole body. I felt the muscles tighten as far as in my toes. I held onto their arms as I doubled over, breathing through it. They were getting worse. The doctor better hurry up or Hope was coming on her own.

At last, we arrived at the bathroom. They helped me onto the toilet and turned around to give me some privacy. I waited. No freaking pee. Now that I was sitting on the toilet I couldn't pee. I tried to squeeze my muscles to try to pee. Nothing but another contraction. *"This is fucking ridiculous,"* I thought that I had just said it to myself. Apparently I used my outside voice because the nurses laughed.

I gave up. I finally stood and tried to pick up the blanket off the floor. I bent over and almost kept going… Suddenly, my horizon line shifted and my world was tipping over. Luckily both nurses grabbed hold of me and helped me back to a standing position. One secured the blanket around my waist and made sure I was completely covered before we ventured back out from the construction hallway and back into the small room. They helped me back onto the table and covered me with the blanket. Then they hung my IV and ran it open wide and hooked up my leads to the monitor. My Dad and Christopher exchanged very unimpressed looks.

The doctor finally arrived with her resident. There were seven people in a room that was maybe 10 by 10 feet. I felt claustrophobic with all eyes on me but felt the medication spill over my body like a heavy veil between me and the rest of the world. I was suddenly very sleepy and even though my eyes were open, everything tracked very slowly and everyone started to blur. The doctor spoke in a matter-of-fact tone, "Okay, guys… we are going to need you to leave the room now. We are going to get started."

My Dad leaned over and kissed my forehead. "I'm scared, Daddy," I mumbled. I don't know if he heard me. I couldn't focus. I turned over to my husband who leaned over, held me, and kissed me. "You're going to be okay. I love you. I love you," Chris tried to comfort me through tears. The doctor gently told him it was time for him to go outside and he released me from his embrace. I wasn't sure if it was the medicine or the fear but I was shaking so hard my knees were literally knocking.

The doctor put her hand on my knee, "Relax, we are on the last leg of this. Just let the medication do its job and try to stay calm, okay? You won't feel any pain. You will feel pressure and movement but you won't feel pain." *'Sure, I have heard that one before,'* I thought. I really didn't know if I was thinking to myself or saying things out loud anymore. To be honest, I didn't care.

She asked me to scoot down to the edge of the table and put my feet in the stirrups. I obeyed, or at least I thought I had. Suddenly, I felt her jerk my hips down to the end of the table. Fear shot through me like a branding iron. She lifted the blanket to be on my stomach and she and the resident sat on their stools. A nurse stood by them, another held an ultrasound wand and another stood up near my head, monitoring my vitals. She was kind enough to hold my hand.

She narrated the first few steps out loud because she told me it would be when I felt the most jerking and pressure. They inserted an instrument and cranked it open wide to expose my cervix. She was pleased with how much I dilated myself and with the help of the bamboo shoots. They had swollen to ten times their actual size to help everything open up. She began removing them, one by one, I felt her grab with forceps to pluck and pull. Twelve times my cervix strained from the pulling then released the shoot and I felt every single one—not in pain per say—but felt the pulling and release. I didn't think it was possible but she then cranked the instrument WIDER and opened my cervix further. It sent a jolt down my legs and severe pain in my belly.

The shock made me gasp. Panicked, I gripped the nurse's hand. I locked eyes with her in desperation, pleading for an escape but I only saw her face. She had mocha skin, beautiful dark curly hair, and burnt sienna eyes. She had smile lines I could see because she gently smiled at me reassuringly. She mouthed, "It's okay," to me over and over and rubbed my hand. Tears streamed down my face as I mourned our baby and feared for my life. Then blackness crept in and I was gone.

I was floating in water, black water with blackness around me. A distant light shone bright white, only enough to illuminate the surface of the water. "This is nice," I thought, "This would be a nice place to die." The tone of my voice wasn't laced with fear, it was a gentle comforting. I don't have to suffer anymore, I can go too. I lay in the black water, not afraid, waiting to die.

That's when I felt an excruciating pain in my chest.

I had passed out and a nurse was vigorously rubbing my sternum with her knuckles to wake me back up. I stayed conscious long enough for her to say, "You can't fall asleep. You aren't breathing when you fall asleep." And the blackness dragged me back under.

I floated in the water. A comforting voice was telling me it was okay. That I didn't have to suffer anymore. I can let go. Chris and Cayden will be okay.

Chris and Cayden.

Chris and Cayden would not be okay if I was gone. I struggled against the black water and felt the burning in my chest again. This time I came out fighting.

I had to stay awake. I had to keep breathing. My eyes searched wildly until I found the nurse's face and held her gaze for dear life. I had to stay awake. I had to focus. That's when I felt a hard pull inside me and a release and then a sharp sound. A sound I had only heard when cutting chicken with poultry scissors. It was the unmistaken sound of scissors on flesh. But whose flesh?

That's when I saw a small, misshapen leg being placed into a metal medical dish. I diverted my gaze back towards the nurse's and sobbed. My baby's body was being pulled apart. That's why they told me I couldn't see her after. Her body would be mangled. I panicked and started to hyperventilate.

"Whoa! Sweetie, you need to calm down and breathe. Close your eyes. Your blood pressure is through the roof and you can't keep going like this," the nurse forcefully cooed. I breathed in and out trying to focus on my breath when I felt another huge pull. I kept trying to breathe but it felt like my insides were being pulled out.

Finally, a release but as I opened my eyes I saw that Hope's body was out.

Only her body.

Like a goddamn horror movie. My baby's body, twisted and contorted from her bone disease, was without a head. "One more pull and we will be almost done," the doctor said, seemingly oblivious that I was witnessing the aftermath.

I stared at the ceiling as I felt one last pull. I was unsure if the pain in my broken heart had exceeded the pressure of the pulling but finally her head was out. I wailed with cries as I saw her sweet little face clasped in between the forceps. It was a primal sound that came from the mother in me. A moan that only comes from being helpless to the demise of your baby. I looked at the wall and closed my eyes, tears painting my face—I was too cowardly to face her. I heard the suction and movement inside me and the ultrasound wand on my abdomen. I fell into the blackness once more.

I think they let me be for a while. The next thing I knew, the medical team was standing, eyes on me and the doctor had her hand on my now blanket-covered knee. "I am so sorry, sweetie. It is all over now. Marsha and Jan will help you get dressed and then you can leave. I would prefer you stay local in case you need us tonight. Do not drive all the way back to Salina, I don't want you to risk a blood clot. I am sorry for your loss," and with that being said, she left the room with the resident and one of the other nurses.

The nurse I had clung to, helped me to a seated position, "How are you feeling?" she asked, studying my face. The room was spinning, my eyes were tracking desperately to find level ground. She must have observed that because she asked me if I was going to vomit to which I mumbled no. We waited and eventually the room came to a halt.

They both took one of my arms and locked them with their own. One of them brought my underwear and yoga pants to my feet and helped me bring them up, placing a pad along the way, because of course I was going to bleed over the next few weeks. Fucking great. One of them gave me a large manila envelope with a teddy bear traced on the cover and out we walked into the lobby where my dad and husband were anxiously waiting. I guess I looked as defeated and drugged as I thought I did. I was coming off of the medication and my mental break of what had happened. I felt unstable as the nurses handed me off to them. I burst out laughing when I almost fell over. I couldn't regulate my emotions and felt myself losing grip with reality when they told Chris and my Dad that we needed to call the funeral home to pick up the remains and pay for the cremation.

I was so weak that my legs started shaking, and I felt like melting putty as they successfully loaded me into the backseat of the jeep and buckled my seat belt. I was completely off my rocker and starting to fade away because of the medication. I giggled uncontrollably. I knew what happened was terrible and I couldn't tell or describe the scene to my Dad and Christopher, so, I just laughed. I had no fucking clue how to process what had happened, so laughter was all that came. My head rolled on the back of the seat as the car turned on our way back to the hotel. I kept rocking back and forth because it felt better than laughing. Finally, we came to a stop.

Christopher woke me. I think that's what happens when you dissociate from your body. I needed to call the funeral home. He couldn't do it. It had to be me. I giggled again. It was perfectly ridiculous that I would have to be the one to call after the procedure and I was clearly broken and high on midazolam. They gave me a phone and a folder with the phone number in it. I laughed as I struggled with the buttons. Finally I hit send and the phone rang.

"Hello, funeral home speaking. How can I help you?" a man answered on the other end of the line. I paused, realizing the gravity of why I was speaking and pulled all my strength together to speak clearly. "Hello. My name is Kelsey Huston. I had to terminate my pregnancy today because of a genetic disease in Overland Park. Will you please pick up our baby's body? I filled out the paperwork to have her cremated by herself." There was a pause before I asked, "What do we need to pay for her to be picked up?" He finally responded, "It will be $260 to pick her up and cremate her remains. Are you able to pay that?" My dad heard it because I had it on speaker and he handed me my mom's credit card. I relayed the card information to him. He said the transaction went through and that he would go pick up her body. I thanked him and hung up the phone.

"Here," I practically threw the phone up front. Even though I was floating high from the medication, I was pissed that two grown men couldn't call the funeral home and made me call them. It wasn't fair. My Dad told us that he was going to head back home because everything was over, it was game day the next day, after all. We said our goodbyes, and I couldn't help but notice the look of deep sadness in his eyes. We exited the car and took the side door into the hotel.

We rode the elevator in silence and made it to the room. I was exhausted and woozy from the medication and still in shock. Whereas, Chris was tired from not sleeping the night before so we climbed in bed for a nap. I don't remember drifting off but I do remember the vivid nightmares, reliving the day all over again. It would be months before I got terror-free sleep again.

I woke up before Christopher did, feeling less woozy but more emotionally raw. It was time to tell people that Hope didn't make it. I couldn't stand one more question about a pregnancy that would never come to term and a baby I would never get to hold. I wiggled my feet in the flip-flops lying on the floor in front of me and silently slipped out of the hotel room so as not to disturb him. I took the elevator downstairs and walked out the side door where we came in hours earlier. I had seen a bench just outside the door and I needed some fresh air in solitude. I sat on the bench and called my mom first to check on my dad. She told me he had just made it home – we felt so overwhelmed that we ended up crying. It was a strange feeling—sympathy from my mom—but it was a relief to cry with someone who knew the truth about what happened to Hope.

My next phone calls were to my Aunt and my Grandpa, I told them simply that the complications of the Osteogenesis Imperfecta Type II were beginning to take their toll and the termination just ended her suffering and our emotional suffering. I missed my Grams, she would know the right words to say to everyone, and would probably make the calls for me or hold my hand while I did or stroke my hair. The story I told Jamie, Sandy, Alicia and Hannah was that the complications had ended her life. Finally, I heard my phone buzz… it was Christopher asking where I was. I replied and headed back inside, up the elevator, and to our room. The door swung open before I had a chance to open it. He emerged from the room and hugged me. I guess he was scared something had happened to me. He pulled back from our embrace and told me that my dad had left us money for food. There was a Chicago style pizza restaurant attached to the hotel, and I could taste food from home. I was still high from the medicine and was starving to death. It had been almost 24 hours since I had eaten or drank anything last so we went downstairs and sat in a booth. The restaurant was empty except for us. We ate, held hands, and intermittently I cried.

We finished our pizza and returned to our room. I don't remember what we watched or what was said, just that I silently let tears stream down my cheeks until I fell asleep.

CHAPTER 4

On Saturday, we picked our son up from Manhattan, Kansas, where he was staying at my sister's house. My parents were at game day with their friends, insisting that we came to their tailgate. There was a snowball chance in hell that I would go to a tailgate after it hadn't even been 24 hours since what I went through. It felt good to hold my son, but the pain in my heart reignited when I saw him. *"Our babies,"* I thought, holding back my tears so Cayden couldn't see or else, he'd get worried. He could tell we were sad, though, and danced in his own four-year-old fashion to the music on his show on TV to lighten up the atmosphere.

On Sunday, Christopher and I spoke in hushed tones in the kitchen. "We need to tell him sooner rather than later," Chris whispered, "I found this idea on Reddit..." *"Great, life according to Reddit,"* my brain flippantly thought, but I genuinely had no idea how to broach the subject with a FOUR-year-old. I was, after all, still bleeding and still processing from the events from the past few days.

The idea was to watch *The Land Before Time*—you know, the movie that starts with cute baby dinosaurs then BAM! Little Foot's Mom dies. The rest of the movie is sweet enough with him intermittently grieving his mom and the instance where he makes a reference to the "Great Circle of Life." Anything is better than some Jesus bullshit and I was fresh the fuck out of ideas so '*Land Before Time*' it was.

Chris and I sat on either side of Cayden and we watched Little Foot's Mom's death scene. All the while, I had tears rolling down my cheeks and I desperately wiped them away. I studied my baby's face. His life would be changed in 20 minutes. I grieved for his excitement of becoming a big brother. I grieved for his big, beautiful heart that had already become entangled with baby Hope. His laughter hurt my chest. I remember how the weight of this discussion felt similar to the weight of when I told Chris I was pregnant with Cayden. Not knowing what would come next, just that our lives would change forever. I remember thinking that it would be the worst day of my life. Boy, did I stand corrected now?!

And just like that, Little Foot's Mom died. Chris paused the movie and we sat in silence for a moment. Christopher started,

"Cayden, you know how Little Foot's Mom went to the great beyond. Well, the baby in mommy's belly, your little sister..." his voice cracked as tears began to flow and I picked up the conversation, "She went to heaven. She's not in my belly anymore... she had to go be in the clouds in heaven." Silence befell upon us as the three of us sat there, staring at each other, while we waited for his little mind to process what we were saying. "My baby sister is in the clouds?" Cayden finally asked. "Yes, in heaven. She had to go up in the clouds." I mustered the courage to reiterate those words. "Can we visit her?" My baby

innocently asked. "No, baby... we can't visit her. She is too far away. How does this make you feel?" "Sad," he began to sniffle, "I really wanted a baby sister here with me." Christopher and I held him together. Chris spoke next, "So did we, bud. I'm so sorry." We just held each other for a while, none of our eyes were dry anymore, but it was alright for we were all together in this. None of our eyes were dry, but it was alright for we were all together in this. When we all calmed down, we turned the movie back on and finished it.

For days after, I would catch Cayden looking out his bedroom window or on our way home from preschool. "There she is! She's in the clouds," he would quietly exclaim and I would fall apart all over again inside.

On Tuesday, I returned to work. Not because I thought I should be there but because I didn't know what else to do. I didn't have any paid time off. Because I was just promoted a month ago and my family needed my share of income. That's what I told myself at least.

The truth was, I had no business being there. My whole soul was broken. I moved through the motions slowly, like my limbs were weighed down by bags of sand. Somehow I still ended up at work two hours early. I would've said that I was the first one there but my boss, Wendy, beat me to the opportunity.

I lazily walked into my office and dropped off my bag before ambling to Wendy's office. I pause before entering her office because for a moment I thought I was not ready for that. I sighed and walked in the doorway.

I didn't even have enough time to speak before the tears started flowing. The truth was, I needed someone I trusted to fall apart in front of. She asked if she could give me a hug and I vigorously shook my head in affirmation. She embraced me and I cried into her shoulder. She asked me if there would be a funeral. I told her no but she would be cremated. I didn't tell her I had been rejected by seven churches already to get her ashes blessed.

More tears flowed when I saw my coworkers, Barb and Amber. Barb actually gifted me her paid time off last week while I was out. I am eternally grateful for that. My family was able to eat that week even though I hadn't earned it by working. They told me they would put everyone straight to voicemail or to Brian because I was still actively crying at the drop of a hat. I am once again thankful for these ladies' discretion because I wouldn't have guessed what happened next.

I don't remember who called first—the funeral home or the clinic—to be honest. However, I got the news that the funeral home had still not picked up my baby, which sent me into a deep hysterical spin.

I shut the door to my office. Whoever had called had hung up the phone. My baby. My Hope. She was still at the clinic, in a box somewhere, and had been for 1...2...3...days! My baby had been shuffled around in a box at the clinic for three fucking days! My fingers raked through my still-wet curls as I suppressed a silent scream. My baby. The baby I wanted, that we loved. My baby was still in a box somewhere like a pair of shoes!

I called the clinic and asked why they had not called for Hope's body to be picked up. They said, "It isn't a procedure for us to call for pregnancy tissue..." to that, I shrieked "My baby!" before they continued, "...to be picked up." I waited for a moment to calm myself down before I said, "But I signed all the forms so I wouldn't have to call." To this, she flatly replied that I still had to call the funeral home. Just like that, the line disconnected.

I called the funeral home and spoke to someone, a young man. I told them that I needed them to pick up my baby, Hope Charlotte Walker, from the hospital as the hospital instructed me to call them. She had been there since Friday. "Please, *please*," I urged, "Please, pick up Hope."

"Ma'am, unfortunately I can't do that. I need the doctor to call me to confirm the death so I can pick up the body," he responded. "They told me to call you, so I am asking you to please pick her body up." "I'm sorry… I can't do that." "Okay, I will have them call you." I hung up this time. My breathing was haggard as I started hyperventilating. I paused and looked at my meager bank account. Enough to make it to Kansas City and back *maybe* if I need to pick up her body myself.

Once again, I called the clinic. I told the receptionist that I needed to speak to Doctor Ryan. She asked me what it was regarding and once again, I explained that I had terminated my pregnancy on Friday and I needed to call the funeral home to pick up my baby's body. She told me that she would get the doctor the message and ended the call.

I sat, curled over my phone, fingers woven tight in my hair, pressing into my temples, rocking back and forth. Minutes passed that felt like hours. Finally, the phone rang, and I checked the caller ID and was relieved to see that it was the doctor's office. I answered, verifying my name and date of birth. "I spoke to the doctor," a nurse on the line began, "she can't call the funeral home, you have to call them." "But I have talked to them and have told your office three times now that you all need to call them." "No, you need to have them call us." My blood boiled and the line disconnected.

I dialed the funeral home one more time. I was going to rip them a new asshole. I asked for the funeral director briskly when a familiar voice came on the line. When he answered, I promptly fell apart. My heart had broken all over again that my baby had been irreverently left in a box somewhere. "Please, *please*," I begged," Please, go get our baby. We wanted her, we love her, please pick up her body." Sobbing racked my body uncontrollably. "What's your baby's name?" he asked in a warm tone. "It is Hope Charlotte Walker. She's at the clinic. Please get her. Her body has been there since Friday. Please, please go get my baby," I pleaded.

"I will leave right now and go pick up Hope," he replied softly, "I will go get your baby." "Oh, thank you," I sobbed, "Thank you so much. We just wanted her so badly and loved her. Thank you for picking up our baby."

I placed my phone on the desk end and waited again. Begging God, begging my passed family for Hope to be received by the funeral director. I willed all my energy, all my heart into begging God and my relatives, in praying for my baby once again. For her protection, for her body to be taken care of because we love her, we wanted her and she was all I could focus on.

20 minutes, 30 minutes, an hour passed, and an unknown number called my phone. It was the funeral director. He had called from his cell phone from his car. He had Hope and was returning to the funeral home. "Oh, thank you so much," a sense of relief filled my chest, "Thank you for picking up Hope." He replied that he was honored to be trusted with her and that he would be in touch soon before he disconnected the line.

I sighed in relief and cried. I laid curled up on the floor of my office and cried. What the fuck was that? Why did they leave her to rot in a box all weekend? I had been like a lioness in a cage with her cub on the outside. I was trapped, unable to reach her, unable to hold her or protect her. Clawing, crying, and begging for her to be cared for. Now that she had been picked up, I collapsed at the bottom of the cage. 11:25—It had been three hours of calling and begging and now that I laid on the floor ready to sleep, I realized that it was time to pick up Cayden from preschool. I picked myself up despite my limbs feeling heavy, and took a deep breath before I opened the door.

FIRE

[PART 2]

CHAPTER 5

By Saturday, I felt weak. I was grasping at my sanity as I sat curled in a blanket on the love seat, while Chris was perched on the couch in our room. Cayden played on the floor in front of us. It was an uneventful day until the doorbell rang. Christopher and I met each other's gaze as we both shared confused looks. We weren't expecting anyone.

Chris opened the door to a very nervous, ashen post officer, "Hi, um, here's your package." She handed Chris a package, staring at the ground and pushing her e-signer in front of him. Chris quickly signed it, and closed the door after thanking her. He turned to face me with the package in his hands and I saw why the post woman had acted so strangely. In big, bold, red letters was a label screaming "HUMAN REMAINS."

Hope's ashes... I didn't expect them to come so soon. He handed it to me and I held it in my hands. Tears welling in my eyes even before I opened the yellow envelope. Once I did, I peeked inside where there was a small white cardboard box with Hope's full name on it. I opened the container to find a tiny plastic bag filled with coarse grey and black ashes, wired shut with a round dog tag attached? Upon further inspection it wasn't a dog tag—it was a death tag— just like the ones you see in the movies. It had her cremation location and cremation number. I cupped the package of ashes in my hands and held them close to my heart. This was all that was left of our baby. Maybe two tablespoons of ashes but at least it was something to hold… to punctuate her death. Tears slipped from my eyes, rolling down my cheeks until they fell into my hands as I held what was left of Hope.

I walked her back to the bedroom where the ornate jewelry box sat on my dresser, and placed the bag of ashes and the death tag inside the red velvet lining. Part of me said, "*She's safe now…*" in an attempt to console my bleeding heart.

"*Now that she, Cayden, and Chris were under one roof with me, they were all safe,*" I thought to myself. Closing the lid of the ornate jewelry box gently, I moved up to the bed and sat on it, all the while staring at the box. I don't know what I was waiting for but I sat sentient for hours staring at the box.

One week after the procedure, I had to go back to the same clinic for a checkup. Christopher and I dropped Cayden off at my parent's house in Manhattan so that he wouldn't have to go in that place or see me go in there. It was a quick check up, the doctor did an ultrasound to make sure that none of the 'tissues' had been left behind that could cause infection. They were also shocked that my bleeding had already stopped. They prescribed antidepressants to help me deal with the emotional stress. Some of those were the ones I had been on before but they also recommended that I go to a psychiatrist and psychologist to process what happened. They just wanted to make sure I had something on board leaving the hospital and birth control that they gave me sample packs of. My legs nervously hopped throughout the conversation and I saw flashbacks of us in those hallways that day and the horror of the events of that day made my heart race. It seemed as if I was reliving the entire experience all over. I was relieved when they let me leave. I half jogged to the car, got in and went to a gas station to go to the bathroom, instead of trying to use the one I had used a week ago... I just didn't want to suffer at the hands of more horrific memories of that unfortunate day.

I was sweating, shaking, and scared but I survived the trip. We got in my car and pointed it West to Manhattan from Overland Park to pick up our son. We pulled into Manhattan and went to a jeweler my mom had recommended. I had been carrying Hope's ashes with me that day. I pulled the ornate jewelry box from my bag and showed it to the jeweler, as I asked, "Can you please engrave Hope's name on the box?"

He looked at the box and thought for a moment before saying, "We can... but it will be tricky on a round surface." I practically begged him to do whatever he could as I removed the tiny bag of ashes from the box and placed them in their original white container. He looked at me with a softened demeanor and asked, "Oh, whose ashes are those?"

I met his gaze, his eyes misty as he already knew the answer, "My baby Hope's ashes. She died last week."

"Oh," he paused, "We will take very good care of this for Hope." He patted the lid of the jewelry box. I gave him my contact information and left.

Climbing into my car, tears falling from my eyes for my tiny baby and her tiny bag of ashes.

The Saturday after we lost Hope, Christopher's parents—Judy and Dwight—came out to Salina to visit us. They brought delicious homemade comfort foods and Cayden was thrilled to have Grandma and Grandpa to play with. I don't think Christopher or I were prepared for what they had brought with them. Several colorful construction paper cards from our nieces and nephews that were tastefully written in crayon, expressing their love and their sympathy for our loss. This gesture from such sweet, innocent children touched my heart as tears welled in my eyes. We read every one and squeezed Cayden a little tighter that night.

Judy and Dwight inquired about the last time we had left the house besides for work to which we replied that we hadn't. They offered to take us to the movies since in Salina tickets are just $4.00. We let Cayden pick out the Minion's movie. Cayden sat between his grandparents and I sat next to Christopher. We were barely past the opening credits when I laid my head on Christopher's shoulder and drifted off to sleep. I didn't have any nightmares that night… indeed a little mercy for me. I guess that having Cayden safe with his grandparents took the energy out of Christopher too because we both awoke with large yawns when the lights came on in the theatre.

The next morning we took Cayden to the park. His giggles filled the air as he played. On the inside, I was sobbing, hurting for his sister who should have been here. I was relieved that he was happy even for this time, we hadn't heard his giggles or his

'Seth Rogen laugh.' Time passed so quickly, and it was suddenly time for them to head back to Kansas City. I wanted them to stay and keep making Cayden smile. A part of me still thinks that if I would have just opened my mouth and asked maybe they would have stayed.

The universe sometimes puts people in our path at the time when we need it. That was the case with Jeff and Wendy Shaw. I had accepted the promotion to come to this job because I adored Wendy, her leadership, and her strong-professional-woman prowess. I had met her husband, Jeff, at the staff retreat on Council Grove Lake before we found out we would lose Hope. He was just a happy, ball of light of a person. In a past life, Jeff had been a genetic counselor and Wendy had offered a couple of times for Jeff to come and talk to Christopher and me. When I was finally ready, she put me in contact with him and one night, after Cayden went to bed, Christopher, Jeff and I sat at our dining room table. I grabbed some notebook paper to take notes because processing information still felt like I was hearing everything underwater.

Jeff met us with a sweet smile and hugs, and sat next to me. He took the paper and pencil from me and explained just a higher level genetics 101 at first. He explained the recessive and dominant genes and how they are passed on. Then onto mutated genes and how they can be passed on. Hope's genetic condition was unique because it is a spontaneous mutation, which means that it wasn't something that was passed down. The reason being that no one with this genetic mutation survives longer than thirty days of life if they live outside the womb because they suffocate from their lungs not developing. It was just a random mutation. It wasn't anyone's fault. No one passed it down and it wasn't anything that I did to cause it. It was just random.

Part of me was relieved to hear that I hadn't caused it but the fact that the 'random' had to happen to our child stung. Jeff met our eyes with warmth while he talked... his tone was immensely kind. I know that the geneticist had explained it to us before but I needed to hear it from someone I trusted and not in the throes of everything that had happened in those short ten days.

The nights when I was home alone were the ones when I felt the most desperate. I sat, staring blankly at the wall. Frozen in flashbacks and grief. On the outside, I looked stoic, whereas, on the inside, I was burning in hell.

My thoughts raced, one flashback after the other. The Midazolam did not do the job it was supposed to. Or my body was too packed with adrenaline during the procedure. Or my high resistance to medications intervened. One thing was certain:

Midazolam was a lie.

The name of the drug sounds fantastical and trippy. It is injected into a patient to take away anxiety, induce sleepiness, and help the patient forget a surgical procedure. While it made me less-ish anxious and drowsy...

I remembered everything.

At first, for the first few hours after the procedure I was out of it. My dad and husband ushered me to the hotel where I slept. I thought I was having a nightmare at first but I was awake. My body shook and that was the first time I was unable to break free.

It was my first flashback. I have had hundreds—maybe thousands ever since. I hear things, the squeak of the cooler for Hope's body and the metallic crunch and snip of scissors on flesh. I see in fervent detail—every gory detail of the surgery.

There is no mercy. I have been punished with this hell for the rest of my life.

CHAPTER 6

I have always struggled with my faith. My paternal Grandmother, who looked after me when I was young, was Jewish (by heritage and religion), and so was my Dad. My mother and her whole family were devout Catholics.

I related the Catholic Church with fire, brimstone, and an angry God. Whenever my Mom forced us to attend church, I felt my skin crawl with the lengthy services that spoke about the crucifixion of their savior, Jesus Christ.

I associated God in the Jewish view with love, freedom, and hard work. At the center of the Jewish religion is hard work. If you live your life by putting all of your efforts into your work and doing *"good"* things, you will be rewarded with the love of God in the afterlife. No, we do not believe in the fire and brimstone of Hell like the Catholics do. Instead, we believe in a stopover—a place for you to work over your sins before you ascend to the afterlife. If you do something truly "evil," you are cast out into the infinite universe or never leave the stopover.

There is a lot of nature versus nurture of the religions that I would need another book to unpack. But for now, let's focus on God in relation to what happened to Hope.

Hope had died just over a month back. I was still fresh with grief, guilt, and the pain of losing a child. I had prayed to God several times over the ten days from when we had found out that there was something wrong to the day she died, but had not prayed since. Anger towards God had begun to set into my heart.

How could he let this happen to our baby? How could he force us to take this option? Why would he make a disease to make a baby suffer like that? I had so many questions and no answers. Yes, it was my belief that God had some explaining to do. Faith-bound family and friends kept saying that God had a plan—there was a reason for it. You know what I think about that?

Fuck God's plan.

Our baby had suffered needlessly, and now our family was suffering from her loss. I watched from inside my hollow shell as my son, Cayden, cried himself to sleep over his baby sister, and my husband mourned the loss of his baby girl, unable to comfort the pain away. I was enraged that a God who was so loving could not do this to the same people whom he loved and looked after. God couldn't do this to a little baby.

I did the only thing I thought I could do… I sought out help. There were a number of support groups in the newspaper, and there was an abortive support group number. I should have just stuck to the damn list the doctor had given me, but I was desperate. I was falling apart, and so was my family.

I called the number and a man answered the phone. I explained what had happened to Hope, and I needed some mental health and faith support. He said he would set up a time for us to meet with him and his pastor to talk. He said, "I'm so sorry to hear what happened to Hope and we will try to help you and your husband the best we can." I was relieved and thought that I had finally found someone of faith to help us grieve.

Boy, was I wrong?

I informed at my workplace that I was going to a doctor's appointment. They usually didn't ask questions after that.

Christopher and I dropped Cayden off at preschool and headed to the church to meet the pastor and the man from the support group. Let's call him Jason.

The light and heat were blinding even though it was the beginning of October when we climbed out of the car. The parking lot was empty, which was normal for a church in the middle of the day during the week. As we approached the front door, my heart started racing. I felt this sudden urge to flee, but I tried to shrug it off. I chalked it up to my fear of *'Jesus People'* from my childhood and told myself that they were going to help Chris and I find comfort.

The pastor and Jason met us at the door where we shook hands and exchanged names and pleasantries. The church smelled like a nursing home, and the musty smell intensified when we went into the pastor's office. It was a small space but enough to fit a desk disheveled with papers, two old red velvet chairs, a wooden coffee table, and a faded green plaid couch. Behind the couch, there was a wall filled top to bottom with books that appeared to be spilling out and had been moved and used frequently as it was evident by the state of the books. Natural light streamed from outside through a large window at the other side of the wall—surely the culprit behind the fading color of the couch.

Christopher and I sat on the couch, close to each other but not touching. The pastor and Jason took their seats in either of the large chairs. "Well, I will get us started," Jason said, "After my phone call with you, Kelsey, I truly cried and found myself hugging my children tighter. I can't imagine the pain you both are going through. I am so sorry." I felt relief in someone else acknowledging the horror we were going through. "I know it is painful, but can you tell us again what happened so that Pastor Mentis can hear it from you."

So, I recanted the cliff notes version of what had happened to Hope. That we had gone in for just a routine anatomy ultrasound, but they had found out something terrible was wrong with our baby. The marathon of pain—mentally and physically—in Wichita and Hope's diagnosis. On our trip to Overland Parkland when we had to terminate our pregnancy and have her cremated. I did not give them details about the termination, just that it happened because I was afraid and had not even told Christopher what had transpired yet.

There was a lingering pause after I finished. I felt a weird shift in energy as the pastor shifted his body language. He had one hand in a fist curled under his chin as I had spoken, but now he leaned forward with his fingers interlocked, eyes on me. Jason mimicked this body language. The intensity prickled up my spine.

"Thank you for telling us your story," Pastor Mentis started, "I am sorry for your loss. I wanted to reassure you that Hope is in a better place now… she has gone to be with the Lord. She is not hurting anymore." He handed me a tissue box as I had been crying.

"Thank you," I said, wiping my cheeks.

"Let's say a prayer for Hope," as trained, we all bowed our heads and closed our hands together, "Lord, please take Christopher and Kelsey's daughter Hope into your kingdom and let her feel no more pain. Please accept her as one of your children and be welcomed into your heart, God. Amen." He concluded the prayer, and we all opened our eyes. Suddenly, his face felt so much closer to mine. "God will not take your sins out on Hope, but you will stand accountable for your sin." I froze, afraid, his eyes still locked with mine. He continued, "Abortion is one of the ultimate sins in the eyes of God. People burn in hell for this kind of sin. I will pray for you and your grief, but you will have to answer to God for your choice."

I sat, mouth agape, stunned at the softness of his tone while he explained the damnation of my soul. Christopher broke the stinging silence with, "We need to go pick up our son from school." The pastor and Jason wished us the best of luck and told us to call if we wanted to do another session.

Yeah. Fucking. Right.

We climbed into the car before I let myself sob. I felt like an awful human being. Guilt for our decision washed over me. We were supposed to receive comfort from the pastor and Jason for our grief, but we had instead received sentencing for my soul. I broke at the thought of God's rejection, and my anger with him swelled. How could God and messengers for him be so calloused to our only option to save our daughter from suffering and having a painful death and save my life? I felt the foundations of my belief in God crack and shake like an earthquake inside of my heart.

As a child, I had learned that God was loving. As a teen, I had experienced a wrathful God through the force of the Catholic Church. Now, God was my judge, jury, and the executioner of my soul. My faith shredded like little pieces of paper. God will take care of my daughter, so at least I had that… but as for me, I might as well just quit while I'm ahead, right? It didn't matter how many youth and adults I helped through the fundamentals of my work, who I volunteered for, what organization I served or how good I was to my surviving son. My soul was going to burn in hell.

I had news for God that I was already burning in hell. I recognized weeks earlier that I sometimes dissociated myself from reality and was lost in the pain and suffering that was my grieving and guilt from not being able to save Hope. Hours and hours of being plunged into a dark, dark space without any end in sight.

CHAPTER 7

After our session with Jason and the pastor, all of my guilt, grief, and flashbacks dialed to eleven. How could I have done this? It felt like my soul was peeling off of my body, that my head and heart could not reconcile what had happened. The visual of Hope's body without a head haunted me. The crying doctor and fighting with the funeral home played like a bad song on the radio in my brain. It was out of control and completely unexpected.

When one would come on, it was like a veil dropped between me and the real world, and the experience played over again, with a higher intensity. I would hold onto a seat or my pants for dear life, shaking uncontrollably, with my eyes tracking. I noticed having sweats sometimes after the episode, as if I had been running in a horror film. Except, it wasn't a horror film, it was my memories in the worst hell form of a replay.

When I would get home at night, I was safe to let them play out and rage over and over again. But there were other times, like at work or while driving, when they would become dangerous.

My work territory was 8 counties large. Driving was an essential part of my job to serve the volunteers and youth in their communities. I couldn't expect them all to come to me when some lived up to an hour and a half away. One early morning, on my way to a little town called Beloit, I had some signs in the back of my care and other promotional materials. As I turned off the highway and onto the country road, the materials shifted, and all of a sudden, a horrible squeaking sound came from the back. It was the foam signs that were responding to each of the broken pavement bumps with a squeak. Just a squeak... a squeak...

SQUEAK

Bam! The veil dropped while I was driving, and I swerved and over-correct. Luckily, I managed to pull over and parked my car on the side of the road. I panted as I fell into the flashback. The squeaking of the foam cooler on the way to Overland Park. The lonely car ride with Christopher, not talking, no music, only the *squeak*. We had packed a small foam cooler in the car as instructed by the funeral director—my mother's friend. He had been very kind to our situation and offered to take care of Hope's body if the clinic did not have procedures in place. The catch: he was in Overland Park, two and a half hours from the clinic, which meant we would have to transport Hope's body ourselves. My baby's body was in a cooler on ice like you do with steak. Luckily, the clinic did have a funeral home they contacted directly, and it never came to that. Still, the trauma of it being one of the two possible options lingered, and the squeak of foam would forever be associated with her death.

Finally, the flashback concluded. I sat behind the steering wheel, holding it tight enough that my knuckles had turned white as I tried to calm my breathing. It was over... I unclicked my seat belt and slumped back on my seat. In a fit of rage and grief, I screamed to the sky as the October wind whipped me in the face. I yanked the signs out of the back and stopped myself before breaking them over my knee. I needed to deliver the signs for work, so I simply disconnected them from the rods and buried them under everything else, weighing them down to prevent the squeaking from continuing. I slammed the trunk shut and raked my fingers through my hair with a deep sigh, and let tears roll down my cheeks. I climbed back in the car, leaving the moment on that dusty road.

<hr>

That night I felt desperate as flashbacks raged and memories of Hope's body without a head, mangled from her disease, tortured me. If it were possible to be dehydrated from crying, I would have been by then. I was spiraling fast. I pulled out the list of three numbers from the clinic and dialed the number for the abortion hotline. A young woman answered and asked if I was suicidal. I lied and said no, and told her that I was just really sad. She asked me what she could help me with that night, and I blurted out everything that happened that day in that tiny, dark room. She intermittently verbalized some *"ohs"* or *"I'm sorrys,"* but overall, it was just word vomit on my part. When I finally finished, she quietly said that she couldn't imagine what I was going through and was sorry for my loss. Then just awkward silence, a really long awkward silence. I sighed and thanked her before hanging up the phone. I didn't feel any better. It felt like I had just unloaded my problems on a teenage volunteer that didn't know what she was doing, didn't know what I had been through or how to respond properly.

I looked at the time, only fifteen minutes had gone by. I still had to wait for several hours until Christopher came home, and I didn't think I could bear the loneliness again, so I called Jamie. To my luck, forever loyal Jamie answered. I asked her if she had time to talk, as I didn't want to bother her if she was busy, to which she cut me off with an "I always have time for you, what's up?"

So, I told her Hope's real story, that we had to terminate the pregnancy and that I was so sorry for lying, but I was too ashamed and scared to tell anyone. I could feel her hug me through the phone as she cried with me and told me that she had no words to express how sad she was for us. She did her best to comfort me and talk me through everything, pouring love into me. Jamie had been my battle buddy at Philmont, and we had seen some shit together. She lives in Minnesota now, but I could feel her climb in the fox hole with me that night and fight off the darkness. Holding off the shadows and the sadness that came with my trauma and grief.

———◦———

I remember the night I made the noise.

Christopher and I had traded off the car, and I sat at home again. I had tucked our sweet four-year-old son into bed and walked down the stairs into our basement like I had every night. Nothing terrible had happened that day. My days were filled with flashbacks, and nights were filled with nightmares. Exchanges with Chris had been strained with indifference like we were ships passing in the night. Neither of us knocked on each other's doors for attention, and no attention was given out. Intimacy in the very basic variety of hand-holding had been absent for weeks. Cayden was my bright spot, excited about learning and full of laughter. Still, I couldn't help but notice how I dimmed his shine that day.

As I put him to bed, he asked me about his sister in the clouds and told me he missed her, and I told him that I missed her too. He asked if he could go to the clouds to visit her, and I told him—choking on my tears as I held them back—that we couldn't visit, and I hoped he wouldn't go there for a very, very long time. His eyes became sad, and he turned over in bed to face the wall. I kissed him on the cheek, gave him a hug, and left the room, closing the door behind me.

I knew I had failed him. I was drowning in my grief, unable to comfort my own child.

What kind of mother was I anyway?

As I took my place on our couch, my mind began to race. I am a mother that killed her baby so that her family could grieve sooner. *'I am a calloused murderer.'* I couldn't comfort the child I have.

"I am a failure."

"I don't feel a connection with my husband anymore."

"I am worthless."

"Why am I trying?"

I scanned the room slowly, looking for a source to my end. An electrical outlet? No, not strong enough. I wanted to draw out my final moments. For the most part, our basement was bare, and I was frustrated until my eyes fell upon something red in our laundry room. The climbing rope—we had bought during our last move—sat coiled in a pile. I walked over, picked it up, feeling the soft texture in my fingers, and I looked up. The floor structure and beams were exposed in this section of the basement. My eyes widened in possibility.

I calculated that I was short enough, and the beam was strong enough for me to hang from if I made a short noose. I began to wrap the rope into a noose, feeling every ring fall into place. Unfortunately, I was very good with knots, so I knew it would hold. I sat on the cold, cement laundry room floor and ran my hands over the noose. I was entranced with the idea of peace, of no longer feeling the weight of my daughter's death, my son's happiness, and my husband's future on my shoulders. Being free to not feel what was expected of me to feel. The ultimate numb. The only way out. I lightly rocked with thoughts of relief and rest when I felt a push from behind.

"What the hell," my trance broke. Our Australian Shepherd was throwing his hip into my back. I thought I was alone in the basement. I had forgotten about the dogs. I gasped when he hit me again. I put the noose in my lap. "What am I doing," I whispered. I shook my head like it was a bad dream and began to weep. The sense of peace and relief had left, and with it, so had my nerves. I was raw as my emotions began to fall out, and I wailed out to the empty space. I found my old hiking backpack and stuffed the noose in there, and stashed it under the stairs. I wasn't ready to let go of it but rather held onto it like a twisted security blanket.

I turned to meet Ranger's face, whose furrowed brown brows seemed almost human. I asked him if he had to go potty, to which he wagged his tail, and his look of concern broke into a goofy panting smile. The moment of thinking he knew what I was doing had thankfully passed. I took him and our other dog upstairs to go to the backyard and met the cold November air.

I stood on our back porch, facing the moon in the moonlight. It was almost full and spilled light across the yard so I could see the dogs, but mostly I looked at the moon. Wondering if Hope was up in the Heaven or if she was with me, if there was life in the spirit after death. Tears pricked my eyelashes, and I held my head in my hands. Shame washed over me. How dare I try to check out Cayden and Chris?

I walked back into the house when the dogs ran up to the door. I set the alarm on my phone to wake me before Christopher got home from work. I then quietly tiptoed into Cayden's room, carefully climbed under his covers into bed, and draped my arm over him. He took my hand in his two small ones and held it to his cheek. I breathed in his smell, felt the smoothness of his warm little hands, and felt my heart kindle in my love for him as I drifted off to sleep.

It was another night in my usual curled-up position on the couch, with grief, guilt, and flashbacks raging. I wept to myself, contemplating ways to end my suffering. There were consistent suicidal ideation undertones in my thoughts that night. I needed a lifeline, someone who understood the dark place I was in because I had lost Hope.

I remembered a friend of mine, Greg, mentioning that he and his wife, Christi, had lost a child. It had been one of those random nuggets that had filed away in my brain from the life-talks we had when we were on work trips. Nothing untoward ever happened, but the talks were always a place of solace in a challenging work climate, with him being several years my senior in life and career.

That night, the memory of one of those talks rang in my ear. I picked up the phone and called Greg, and when he didn't answer, I texted. I broke down that we had lost Hope and that I was struggling and was reaching out because I wanted to talk to Christi—mom to mom—as someone who had been in my position… kind of, anyways. He could tell I was hurting and relayed that she would call after they got home from dinner.

"Okay," I said to myself, "I can hold on until then." I paced, rocked, and snuggled my dogs. It wasn't long before a Columbia, Missouri number appeared on my phone, clearly Christi. I took a deep breath and answered the phone.

Her always kind voice answered. She had me explain what happened to Hope, which I did—for the most part, I just left out the termination part and said that we had lost her. I needed help, and I couldn't handle rejection or pity that night. I could feel her soften further as she listened. I then asked her to tell me the story of their baby, Summer, who had been born too soon with her own challenges. Sweet Summer fought hard to stay with her mother and father, but unfortunately, she succumbed and became an angel. She repeated to me a phrase I would keep in my heart, *"Whenever someone asks me how many children I have, I say two, but I always quietly whisper to myself that I have three."* I cried with her, echoing the same absence in my soul. She advised me to seek out counseling right away and to keep myself busy. "I picked up crafting, all sorts of hobbies to keep myself from getting too quiet with the grief," she told me. "Crafting? I love crafting," I responded through the mist of my grief. She then reassured me that I should move through the grief how I need to, and the fact that it will change with time. But, unfortunately, those hours would feel like they were dragged on.

Christi told me to call her anytime I needed to talk, and that I didn't need to be alone or ashamed of my grief before we hung up the phone. The suicidal thoughts had subsided. I looked at the clock, and I still had two hours until Christopher came home. I walked into the laundry room and dug my craft boxes out of the pile of still-packed belongings from the move. I ran my fingers over the ribbons, beads, and paintbrushes. I examined each one for the crafting potential that I had kept it for. Ideas of creation populated my brain as I began arranging, organizing, and making lists of supplies I needed for pictures. I let myself dive into crafting and artwork and take a reprieve from my pain.

⸺⸺◦⸺⸺

My appointment to see the psychologist was at 6:00 PM. I felt guilty for making her stay for what was indeed an after-hours appointment. I was also afraid from my previous counseling experience. I had tried to receive grief counseling from a church to only be told I was going to hell and a psychiatrist wouldn't see me unless I started psychotherapy. My faith that a therapist would help me without any kind of judgment was low, and my hope for crawling out of the dark place that I had found myself in was even lower. I honestly didn't believe that I would ever be just okay again. I don't think I had really smiled since I got hammered at a bar right after Hope died. I had laughed, but it was at random, awkward times, and it wasn't something I could control. Someone said something even a little funny, and my body convulsed, and I laughed as I had just discovered Jim Carey. It was scary to not be able to control my emotions.

Chris noticed that I was having trouble keeping it together. After one too many nights of sobbing when he came home, he offered to contact therapists for me to get some help. I agreed. He found a private practice therapist that night, messaged them, and left a message on their voicemail. Someone responded right away that they had an opening and would see me two days later if I could just hang on until then. I wasn't going anywhere. I was stuck in my slippery damp darkness.

The waiting room of the psychologist's group was nice enough. The furniture was wicker and had tranquil blue cushions, and the lighting was soft. Everything about the waiting room was calming, great for crazies like me. Two locked combination-code doors separated the waiting room from the therapy rooms. I rang the doorbell as instructed on the wall to let them know I was there and waited.

I didn't wait long before a woman came out of the locked door to meet me. She looked like she was in her 30's. She had long brunette hair and black-framed glasses, casually dressed in leggings and a long tunic shirt. She identified herself as Allison and asked if I was Kelsey, to which I responded in affirmation. Allison invited me back to her office.

The lighting was low, with a few lamps decorating the tables. I sat on her blue settee, and she sat on one of the two opposing orange chairs. Colorful paintings dawned on the walls, and in the corner sat some toys. Another calming room for crazies like me.

"So, your husband reached out to us with some concerns for you and explained a little bit about your situation. But why don't you tell me why you are seeking out therapy today, Kelsey?" Allison started.

"I had to terminate my pregnancy because our daughter had a very rare genetic condition. I haven't been able to keep it together since then. I know I need help, and I did try going for counseling, but they told me I was going to hell, so I stopped trying. If you want to be my therapist, you need to be okay with me talking about abortion because I can't get better if I am not honest about what happened to her," I blurted out. I was fast to get it out because I couldn't hold it in anymore. I studied her face for hesitation, pity, or offense. She held steady with her kind smile. I was impressed.

"I am okay with abortion, and it sounds like you are hurting deeply about it, and you are grieving your baby. I am glad that you are seeking out help. I need to ask you some basic intake questions, and then we can talk more about that. Is that okay?" I skeptically agreed. I answered her basic questions about my mental and physical health history. She asked me if I was feeling suicidal then, and I told her that I wasn't. It was the truth. At that very moment in time, I was not feeling suicidal.

It finally came time to talk about Hope, and I felt like bolting. I was afraid to let out what had happened in that small, dark room that day. Allison reassured me it was okay and still took my time with a kind smile on her face, and I wondered if that smile would still be present after I told her everything.

So I told her everything. I started with us finding out we were pregnant the same day I got a promotion, our move, and how excited we were for the baby we were trying for. Then I explained the ten days from the first ultrasound determining there was something wrong with our baby to our day in Wichita up to the day of the termination. I studied her face again. She had been writing but was unwavering with her kindness all the while I talked. I took a deep breath and explained what had happened in that clinic and in that small, dark room.

When I finished, I inhaled, studying her face for horror, shock, or disbelief. Her smile was soft, and her body language remained unchanged. I was impressed, and I let out my breath. She told me what I had been through was tragic and traumatizing and that she was so sorry that it had happened to me. She made me realize that we didn't have a lot of time left, but it sounded like I had been holding in that silent scream for a while and it must feel good to finally have it out. I mentally checked myself as I felt like I had literally deflated. My shoulders rounded and my elbows were on my knees, while my head was tilted towards the ground. Yes, I had finally let it out to someone who didn't flinch, and I felt the weight of the world shift—not off my shoulders but supported by another.

She told me that she wanted me to come back on Thursday to do more of the standard intake questions. I told her I couldn't afford to come back, and she just told me not to worry about it, and I needed to come back.

I came back on Friday and twice a week for a month to get my thoughts stable until I was able to get in to see the psychiatry department at the hospital. She diagnosed me with depression and anxiety with a chief complaint of Post-Traumatic Stress Disorder.

CHAPTER 8

Every year, the Walker's get together for the "Walker Family Fall Festival." All four brothers and their families gather at Dwight and Judy's house for the occasion, before heading off on a hayride in the back property, bob for apples, and paint pumpkins. It truly is a beautiful family tradition with just the right touch of chaos because, at the time, there were 13 grandchildren from baby to eleven running around. The bond between the cousins and brothers, retelling old stories about each other, and the sisters-in-law shepherding the children, cooking (as much as Judy allows), and catching up.

This was the first family fall festival after Hope died, and the wound was still excruciatingly fresh. One thing I had avoided to this point was seeing siblings together. It was another level of grief that I had not brought myself to face—the pain of seeing Cayden without his sister and everyone else with theirs. It wasn't fair! To make matters worse, one of the families had a young baby that would be impossible to not associate with Hope.

When we got to Christopher's parent's house, I sat at my usual station on the couch. So far, so good, and honestly, I was okay until the family with seven children arrived. They all came in and spread out throughout the house and backyard, some making their way into the living room to hug me, which was the sweetest as always. However, I was not prepared for one of them to just plop their baby brother right in front of me on the carpet. He stared at me, and I stared back. His glassy big blue eyes and sweet face, so innocent. I felt myself start to shake, and the veil rolled on. Hope's mangled body flashed before my eyes—her tiny face and the snipping sound pierced my ears. I held onto the old plaid couch, bracing myself, tears running down my face. When it began to subside, I jumped to my feet and caught Christopher long enough to tell him that I couldn't do this and did what I had already planned—evacuated to my Aunt's house.

I climbed in the car and drove down the street to her farm, passing the gate, the horses, and the always vigilant llama, Puppy. When I entered their apartment adjacent to their barn, I was greeted by the menagerie of bulldogs and my Aunt's boyfriend. My Aunt and I had prearranged that I would come over for just a couple of hours if things got too much to handle. Well, it had, so I plopped down on her couch and watched some HGTV with them. I talked about what had happened and cliff notes about my struggles with some things since Hope died, and they listened and supported me.

Eventually, Christopher texted to ask me to come back up to the house. The text briefly mentioned how things were winding down, and he was worried about me, so I made my way back to the Walker's house. The house was empty, everyone was out back, so I took a deep breath and stepped out onto the back porch. There was an interesting spectacle unfolding. Michael had backed up his car into the yard and was unloading a small tree off the back. The other brothers were a mixture of helping and herding the children away from the car. One of them shouted to me, "Where do you want your tree?" I looked back at him confused, whereas, Sarah and Genny looked at me with embarrassment, quickly walking over to me. "We got you a tree for baby Hope. Where would you like it planted?" I began to softly cry as I had not expected this from them because most families had avoided talking about Hope at all costs. We chose a spot that could be seen from the dining room table, so we could easily look out and check on it. They called over all of the family to stand in a circle around the tree, and Christopher's brothers—Sam and Carol—who were pastors, took turns saying a prayer for baby Hope. Christopher and I stood in the middle of the circle holding Cayden, next to our tree. I thanked them as this was the closest we could have for a funeral for her. We received long hugs from each one of the Walker clan, and I felt my heart flicker, being surrounded by love.

⸻∘⸻

My mother had been uncharacteristically supportive since Hope died. Days earlier, I had buckled my son, Cayden, into her purple jeep at my office. I stayed up late to put up Christmas decorations so that the angel tree would be up in time for Giving Tuesday so that youth in need would get what they needed for Christmas.

We had a weird Thanksgiving. As we were about to leave, my mom gave me a strange look while I was loading Cayden into my car. She called me on our drive home.

She told me she was concerned. When they picked up my four-year-old Cayden, he had some very grown-up things to say. It wasn't cuss words or inappropriate things, but I needed to get myself together because I was affecting him. I asked her what he had said, and after some badgering, she finally told me.

On the way to her house, Cayden had asked her more than thrice to take him home. Even when they arrived at her house, he asked her to take him home. She finally asked him why to which he replied, "My Mommy needs me." She told him that I was okay, and he burst into tears, "She's not okay! She is sad! She needs me to take care of her! My Mommy needs me!"

My heart broke for my Cayden baby. I asked her what she told him. She told him that he needed to take care of Cayden and be happy for Cayden. That his mom was a big girl, she could take care of herself.

"You have to pull yourself together," my mom pressed, "Cayden is so good, but he is just a little kid. I love you, but you need to pull yourself together."

"Thank you for taking him this week, mom," I replied curtly. I was angry and ashamed that I had put so much weight on a four-year-old's shoulders.

⸻◦⸻

I had been dreading Christmas as we were broke from medical bills and student loans and just not having money, period. My Aunt had gifted us Gram's old tree, though, so we would have our own Christmas tree for the first time ever. We used decorations such as pearls, lights, and Philmont signs from our wedding to adorn the branches and bought a case of ornaments and a star for the tree. Cayden helped decorate the bottom-half of the tree the best way he could. So while Chris was at work, I would stare at the tree now instead of the blank wall, willing Hope to be with us still to no avail.

One night, a package showed up at our doorstep from Amazon. I was confused, I hadn't ordered anything, but it was addressed to me. I pulled a box from the wrapping, and on the gift, the receipt read, "For Hope. All my love, Jamie." I removed the gift receipt to uncover an ornament I had added to my wish-list just a few days ago. It was a pair of angel wings with a blue orb that read HOPE gives us wings to fly. I knelt on the entry floor, removed the ornament from the packaging, and held it to my heart. *"Something for our angel baby for the tree,"* I sobbed. She would be with us for the holidays. I called Jamie and thanked her. She was my Phil-Sis, and I truly had needed that.

When Christopher arrived home that night, we took the ornament together and placed it near the top of the tree. That way, we thought, Hope could watch over us for Christmas.

That Christmas weekend, we traveled to my parent's house for Christmas Eve till next morning and to Christopher's parent's house for Christmas dinner. At each house we stopped at, we carried the ornament with us and placed it near the top of the tree so that she was with us no matter where we were. We also brought Hope's ashes with us. I just couldn't bear the thought of having her be alone on Christmas, and neither could Chris. No one said anything to us and let us be with tears and all as we moved through the holiday in mourning.

Hope's due date was January 26th, and my birthday was January 28th. My heart struggled in separating the two. I couldn't stop thinking that my forever baby in the clouds would never be with us and that I would continue to breathe another year on the earth without her. I had thought for months about getting a tattoo for her. Maybe a wishbone? The symbol for osteogenesis imperfecta? No. Angel wings? No.

On her due date, I held the paper with her tiny footprints, the length of a quarter each, in my hands. This is what I needed tattooed on me. To punctuate how small and innocent she was and how loved by her mother and father she was, just like any baby. I wanted more to it, though, something for me. I settled on the date that she came to us and died. The day my life would never be the same.

Forever changed.

My friend from work recommended a tattoo artist in town that had done some work for her. I took the recommendation, set up the appointment, and just a couple days after my birthday, I sat on the couch in the entry wave of the tattoo shop. I explained to my artist what I needed to be done, where and the cliff notes version of Hope's story. A mixture of sadness and reverence misted in his eyes. He agreed, had me double-check the design, and brought me back to the chair. He shaved the back of my neck lightly and placed the roman numerals right under my hairline. He then placed each of Hope's feet staggered as if they were walking up to my neck behind my ear. It was perfect.

He didn't ask me many questions. Instead, he let me get into my zone. I know that the back of the neck and back of my skull should hurt, but the headspace I was in, doing this for Hope, I felt the buzzing but no pain. I even had my teeth rattle as he moved higher onto my skull, but again no pain came. My grief and pain overshadowed my senses, and I sat like a rock as he finished. When I turned to meet my artist's eyes, he had a sombre composure and charged me less than half of what he quoted me. I was thankful for the compassion he had shown me, one parent to another, and would never forget the memorial he gave me for my daughter.

BETRAYAL

[PART 3]

CHAPTER 9

My little brother was born without a ventricle and with several holes in his heart. While he survived, he couldn't play sports or do most activities that all the other boys could at the risk of triggering a tachycardia episode. My mom got him involved in the safest activity she could think of—Boy Scouts. He had a normal experience like most boys the first several years, but in August of 2005, our whole world changed. Hurricane Katrina hit New Orleans, and while it was hundreds of miles from our Chicago suburb, it meant our dad had to go to New Orleans for recovery efforts. He established temporary buildings for natural disasters like hospitals and housing. Our dad was gone for 250 days that year to help with the recuperation of the city, which turned into years. That meant my mom was on her own for all that time with three teenagers, my younger brother and sister, and myself.

My sister and I were still too young to be left at home for an entire weekend by ourselves during that time. So, when George needed to go on a camp out for Boy Scouts, we all had to go. My mom had to go by default, and we had to be along for the ride.

I loved it. We would camp, hike, fish, and there were no other girls, so NO high school drama. I grew up around these guys, so they were all like brothers to me. Even the Council professionals came to know us by name because we went to EVERYTHING. Wayne practically watched the three of us grow up. This love of scouting led me to work at Cub Scout summer camps in high school. I learned leadership and how to work with people of all ages and creeds.

When it came to my freshman year of college, I had a decision to make. I could go work at the usual council camp like I had done for years and live at home. Or I could go to New Mexico to a high adventure camp that I had never been to before with a job "to be determined" and see what comes of it.

I chose adventure.

I had a four-day turnaround between my last college exam and my flight to Albuquerque. Enough time to drop all of my college stuff at home, pack and shop for a sturdy pair of hiking boots and maybe one sleepover with a perturbed best friend (who was distraught that we wouldn't have the summer together, and I was too. But I could feel this pull for adventure edging me forward). Time flew faster than a snap of my fingers, and I was on a plane departing Midway, with a duffel bag in tow, which was big enough to fit my body in.

It wasn't long before I looked out the plane window and saw the mountains from above for the first time, and couldn't help but have my mouth agape. They were beautiful, god-like titans that rose from the earth.

When we finally landed, I picked up my duffel from baggage claim and walked out to be embraced by the dry, desert heat. I waited for my bus to camp, which was four hours north of there. It was a very inconspicuous airport van, the driver spoke broken English and showed me where to put my bags. She was a sweet Hispanic woman, in her 50's and about my height. All I remember from the ride is that it was long, and we went on the back roads instead of the highway… was there even a highway there? I didn't know. I was in completely unchartered territory with this trip. She could have been taking me South instead of North, and I wouldn't know other than the sun. The second thing I remember about the ride was that she was trying to set me up with her son. I was using all of the Spanish I learned in high school to fill in the gaps in her English. Again, she could be taking me home to her son, and I wouldn't know. Awareness of my unknowing prickled up my spine. I just needed to keep my eyes open, which was hard since I had been traveling since 4:00 am.

The bus ride took ten hours. Not four... not six... Ten. Hours. When we finally arrived at the camp, it was pitch black other than the starlight that vaguely illuminated two adobe buildings. The bus driver helped me unload my duffel, pointed at one of the buildings, and took off in her bus. The darkness was ominous, and I could feel my unknowing prickle again.

A tall man emerged from a door. I didn't see but heard him slam the door behind as he entered. I guessed that the bus arriving woke him, "Hi, I'm Nick, you know the arrival is between eight and five, right?" His voice broke. He was just a college kid like me, giving me a lecture about being in after-hours like he was my father lecturing me about curfew.

My wild showed.

I popped my hip to the side and put my hands on my hips and let him have it. Respectfully, of course. "I wish I could have been here then. At 4 am, I was in Chicago. At 1:00, I was in Albuquerque, and I have spent the last ten hours on a bus that I am certain has not had its struts or shocks changed in at least 15 years. Now I am exhausted, if you can point me to a tent, I will bed down, and we can both get on with our night."

Now it was his mouth agape. I guess he wasn't expecting that much sass at that time at night from such a small package. He gained his wit, "Where will you be working this summer? I will just take you to that tent city." "I don't know, I got a phone call, and Owen said he would figure out where I go when I get here." "Well, I guess you can go to a female tent city for now, and in the morning, you will need to pack up your things and meet with Owen to find out where you belong." "Thank you, I appreciate it." I reached for my duffel, but hc beat me to it. He swung it up on his back like a backpack and used a headlamp to guide the way.

We passed a shower house on our way into the tent city. Rows and rows of canvas platform tents illuminated under the stars. It was silent except for our footfalls in the gravel. We arrived at a tent near the end of the row. He opened it, revealing two cots, a locker, and a single light bulb hanging from a wire strung up to the tent frame. He slid my duffle onto the tent floor. I thanked him, climbed into the tent, and velcroed it shut.

A sudden gust of wind made all of the walls of the tent bow inward. Awesome. I hadn't noticed the wind until now and how cold it was. I fished my sleeping bag, pillow, yoga pants, and sweatshirt out of my bag. I made so much haste getting into bed that I forgot to turn off the light bulb. It was far too cold to get out of my sleeping bag by then, and to be honest, the wind was so harsh and I was so alone I was apprehensive about turning it off anyway. The wind blew harder, and the tent flexed inward, even on top of me. I gritted my teeth. It was going to be a long night. The hours painted away as I slipped in and out of sleep. One thought always came to mind in my waking time:

What the hell was I thinking?

When my phone alarm finally went off, I took out my shower stuff, pulled back the canvas flap of the tent, before stepping into the cool morning air. I wasn't prepared for what was waiting for me outside. Mountains rose for miles around me. I had never seen mountains so close before. I truly felt like an ant among giants. I whispered to myself, "What have I gotten myself into?"

I fell head over heels in love with the place. The sights, the people, and the wildlife. I came back three more summers and held three positions there, ending my time as a search and rescue driver. I had met Hannah, Jamie, and my husband, Chris, and so many others that touched my heart. Mama Sandy filled a special place in my heart—a void that was there since my grandmother passed away—and still sends care packages for our babies. She was the one who I called and cried with when Hope was dying. I owed her and Larry more than I could ever give them.

Scouting had always had a special place in my heart, but it became part of me after my summers at Philmont and fuelled my passion for the outdoors. When I graduated from college, just seven short months after Cayden was born, I held a degree in Fisheries, Wildlife, and Conservation Biology with a minor in leadership studies.

I applied to work for the local area council in Salina, Kansas, to be a district executive. How different could it be, right? The answer was—very different. It was fundraising and recruitment focused, with camping on the side. At first, I was disappointed, but after truly understanding the missions behind the work of not only the Boy Scouts but also non-profits at large. I understood and embraced the purpose behind the work.

After some travelling and some moves, I ended up promoted and back in Salina, Kansas, as a Senior District Executive. It wasn't an accident. I always wanted to go back and adored Wendy as a strong female role model. I wanted to learn more from her, so when she offered a position, I accepted.

When we returned to Salina in July of 2017, it was with fully open arms by the professionals and volunteers alike. Cayden picked up his surrogate grandparent role with Dennis and Nancy as we had never left. Even when Hope died and post-traumatic stress set in, I never felt like my job was threatened.

That all changed in November.

The weird thing about the hierarchy of the Boy Scouts and most of corporate America is that when one person retires, it sets off a chain reaction of promotions. Well, some big wig at the national office retired, and another got promoted. He was pulling Wendy up to be on his team. Don't get me wrong, it was a huge win for Wendy and women "in the movement," as they said, but for me, personally, I was crushed. I had come back to Salina to work for her, and she had been a safe place during the worst moments of my life. I meant this in the most supportive and polite way possible—what the actual fuck? She wouldn't leave the office until January, but the time that she did have left, she spent with one leg on each side. Again, understandable, but it didn't make my grief and struggle any easier.

When she finally left to be in Texas full time, Richard became our full-time point of contact for projects, though he spent very minimal time in Salina. Brian and I did our best hustling along with fundraising and everything else. What scared me was Richard had become very Manhattan-area-centric, and everyone else got kicked to the side. I was still mentally struggling to transition with medication, and I tried my best to ration it away as my anxiety, but others in the office picked up on it too.

Eventually, in February, Kevin, the new boss, was hired, but at that point, Richard was already off the chain with kicking the rest of us around. I couldn't imagine the narrative he told about the rest of us outside of Manhattan was positive. Luckily, despite the drama, I got my wish to go to Philmont Scout Ranch for enrichment training in March.

I drove for nine hours out to Philmont by myself in a rental car. Reliving some of my old haunts and staying at a friend's house the night before training. It was freeing to leave Salina and reground at Philmont. Every morning I woke and inhaled the mountain air deeply, absorbing as much as my HOmE that I could. A week went by way too fast, and on the last morning, I woke early and went to the reservoir.

It was cold, but I took off my shoes to feel the sand under my feet. The sunrise reflected off of the water, dancing with the wind. The last time I was here, I screamed at the sky, unleashing wilderness in me. That morning, I felt the weight of the world on my back, and so I let it crush me. I fell to my knees, hands holding my face, sobs rolling over my body. This grief, this trauma, this life was too big for me. I wasn't strong enough. I wished to return to the simpler times when getting lost in a storm and staying in a tepee at a place called the Snow Mansion was life and adventure.

When I cried myself out, I climbed back in the car and drove the nine-hours back home. Feeling sand-filled bags on my shoulders with every mile.

How would I survive my life?

CHAPTER 10

I met Joe when we were kids in high school. I dated his best friend at the time. But after that phase in my life, Joe and I had remained good friends with minor bouts of being more than that. He had been a horseman at Philmont so he understood the love for the New Mexican backcountry that I harbored. Christopher was not his biggest fan but was as happy as I was when he found Mara. The fiery red-head he had always wanted and he finally asked her to be his wife.

It was unexpected to get a message from him one night as it had been since before Hope died that we talked. Part of their marriage counseling was to have married couples write them letters with advice with what they wish they knew when they got married. I was hesitant due to the distance that Chris and I had been at because of our tragedy. But maybe that was the lesson I had to share...? Once I sat down, the words came flooding out:

Dear Joe & Mara,

Thank you for trusting me to write you a letter on your journey to getting married. While I am no expert, in the short two years that Chris and I have been married and the last seven we have been together, we have learned a lot. My letter won't be all sunshine and brunches like some newlywed letters may be. But I hope that you will be able to take a lesson into your marriage; you won't have to learn the hard way!

Chris and I's marriage didn't happen in a traditional fashion and we have had some very painful growing pains because of that. What has been beautiful to observe is how love is fluid. You don't necessarily love your spouse the same way you did when you shared your first anniversary or even the same way you did last week. That doesn't mean that your love necessarily diminishes or rapidly grows. The way it feels changes and just like all liquids do, it changes to fill the shape of its container. The love I felt for Chris when he was going hungry in college and I would bring him food was different than when he proposed. It was different when we found out we were pregnant—a big reason I put off marrying him for four years. I knew that our love fit in us as a couple... but did it fit in us as a family? Over the time, it grew to fill that shape and we shared it with Cayden, who changed everything all together. Accept that your love is fluid and can fill the container you put it in. Just make sure that it is strong, and selected with care and safe.

Now for the hard part…

If there is one piece of advice I could give any couple above anything else it would be to turn to each other. This doesn't mean the "don't cheat on each other" kinda turning away. I mean, when tragedy strikes your marriage, whether it is the death of a loved one, an illness, an accident or anything that devastates one or both of you… just turn to each other. Turn in to each other for support every time. If you don't, it will create a chasm between you two that will be hard to rebuild that bridge to each other. We have learned this the hard way. We lost our daughter Hope at 20 weeks in September this year to a lethal genetic disease. It was devastating to lose her and the pain in grief of losing a child is unbearable. What's even more painful is that Chris turned away to heal on his own and left me in my grief… what has now developed into post-traumatic stress disorder from her death. It isn't all Chris' fault, though. I stopped reaching for him and truly everyone when no one wanted to talk about our daughter.

I wish I could say that one day there was an epiphany and we came back together and everything is amazing again. It's not. So much love and trust was lost in the void created from turning away from each other. I know it will take us years to recover, if we do recover. We love each other and our son Cayden and it is worth the work. But there has been so much that would have been avoided if we turned to each other.

Turn to each other. Hold them even if they say they are okay. Ask them about the pain they are feeling. Ask them open-ended questions. Validate their pain. Never ask or tell them they should be over it by now. Never underscore their pain. Do the little things—the laundry, a cup of coffee, a kiss on the forehead, or a sweet little surprise in their day. These will keep you bonded when the lattice starts to fray.

Turning to each other is not just about the bad stuff. It's about the good stuff too. Celebrate each other when you accomplish your goals. Every success is a success for you as a family. When one of you moves forward you both do. Don't ever forget that. Do not be jealous, resentful, or descendant of each other's success. You have chosen each other as partners to live with side by side. Lift each other up in excitement! The achievements are achievements for your whole family. Be the first one they want to call and brag about that promotion at work!

Heavy stuff? I know... but truly, appreciate the beauty you see in each other as your love changes. Love one another, support each other, and above all, turn towards each other. Joe and Mara, I know you two love each other and I cannot wait to see you on your wedding day. Don't forget to incorporate your love for dance, adventure, and the romance you have developed into the rest of your lives!

See you in October,

Kelsey Walker

CHAPTER 11

When I found out I was pregnant with Ember, I was terrified.

I had been on an oral form of birth control, and even though my husband and I had sex twice since we lost Hope, there I was, staring at two blue lines making a plus sign. I remember blinking several times as though if I closed and opened my eyes hard enough, it wouldn't be true. I sat on the side of the tub, mortified. I couldn't go through another pregnancy as I did with Hope. My mind couldn't handle it, and I sobbed at the thought.

Everyone has heard of the expression "when it rains, it pours," right? Well, my work had taken a turn for the worse with the addition of a new boss. My once caring and encouraging direct supervisor had been tearing me a new one for weeks since he had arrived. Coupled that with needing to cancel a big event due to an impending ice-Apokolips, and he was all fire and brimstone on me. To make things even better, our gas was going to be shut off the next day because neither my husband nor I could afford to pay it until the following

Friday, when we got paid. So my family was going to freeze, and I was going to get my ass torn up for trying to keep people safe that weekend.

I cleaned myself up and stored the test in my sock drawer for when Christopher came home. I was on edge until then. Cayden had gone to bed, and the flashbacks had crept in. My fear of this pregnancy was taking a hold of my mind. I was shakily preparing for tomorrow's staff meeting with my bosses and trying to figure out the best way to keep my family warm that weekend. Especially, when the temperatures were supposed to drop by 60 degrees with no heat in the house.

I had concluded that since I was going to Manhattan for the meeting, Cayden and I would just stay the night with my parents, and Christopher could come that night or the following weekend. In the meantime, a few of our friends, including Brian and Chris' boss, let us borrow a couple of portable heaters to keep us warm over the week until we got the heat turned back on. We were lucky to have friends who cared about us.

Chris confirmed the plan with me, and we were all set. Now all I had to do was wait three more hours for him to come home from work.

I paced, I rocked, and I shook while counting down the hours. Flashbacks raged. Fear, frustration, and disbelief crossed my mind, and I checked my sock drawer to make sure the test was still positive. Yep. Still positive! Finally, at 11:47, he came home.

Chris came into our room, surprised to find me upstairs instead of my usual spot on the couch downstairs. "Everything okay," he asked. "Just sit down on the bed. We need to talk," I instructed. He did so, a look of worry crossed his face, "What's wrong?" I retrieved the test from the sock drawer, sat down next to him. Without waiting for another second, I just blurted out that I was pregnant, showing him the positive test, before I burst into tears. He said, "Okay, so what do you want to do?" To which I was confused. What did he mean by that? I told him that I was scared this baby would have the same disease that Hope did and I couldn't handle going through that again. "I know," he replied softly, "It is going to be okay. Let's get you checked up soon and try to find out now rather than later if this one has the same issue Hope had." I agreed, and he embraced and held me for a moment before going into the other room to get some dinner.

———◦———

The same week I found out I was pregnant, there was also an ice storm of epic proportions looming for the weekend that we were supposed to have a camporee with the Boy Scouts. I made the tough call to cancel the camporee. People threw fits, but I simply told them it was a safety issue. If someone had driven on the ice and got into an accident on the way to the camporee, I would have never forgiven myself. If it had been snowing, fine-I would have schlepped myself out there—but I and several other event organizers across the mid-west canceled events to keep people safe.

After I made the call, my husband told me we were going to lose heat. We had got too far behind and couldn't pay it until the following week when we got paid. We scrambled, reaching out to friends to get space heaters to warm the house, and tried to insulate the best we could. For the most part, we managed, but it was freezing outside.

That Friday, I had a staff meeting in Manhattan at the Kansas State Alumni Building. I was shaken from my personal life, but everything with work had been okay, I thought. When we went through awards, I noticed four of our categories were missing and spoke up, to which Richard yelled and painted me into a corner in front of the rest of my coworkers and my still-new boss, Kevin. Quiet tears slid down my face when I made eye contact with him, rose to my feet, walked from the room, and went to the restroom. I went to the bathroom stall, curled up in a ball, and cried. My job had always been my solace, but now it had become a shark tank. Our heat was off, and now I was pregnant again while I still mourned our daughter Hope. Flashbacks clouded my brain, and I rocked my body, still glued to the ground.

I didn't know how long I was in the bathroom, but my flashbacks and tears eventually stopped coming, and I returned to the room. Little did I know that Richard was just getting started. For months after, I was threatened and demeaned in front of Kevin. I wasn't sure what kind of dominant point he was trying to prove, but he proved it.

<hr>

We moved into a new house in June. The landlord was weird, but it was beautiful. I couldn't wait to light the stone fireplace in the winter. Chris still worked nights, but this house felt like a clean slate compared to the basement in which I had spent endless hours suffering. I had snuggled in for bed after a long day at camp in Abilene when I woke up by the alarm. Something was wrong. I went to the bathroom and felt wet. I sat down on the toilet, and dark blood *poured* from my body. No. No, no, no, no. This can't be happening. More blood came. I called Christopher in a panic and told him to come home soon, as I was bleeding and losing the baby. I placed a pad in my underwear, put on a sports bra, and went to wake Cayden. He sleepily did as he was instructed. He was such a good little boy. Chris got there a little too fast, and we loaded into the car. Christopher called Brian and told him that we were miscarrying and begged him to meet us at the hospital, which he did.

Flashbacks of Hope raged around me as Chris drove. I whimpered and shook in fear. Brian met us at the hospital, and I hugged Cayden tight as Brian took his hand and led him out to the truck. We were lucky to have him, Lisa, and their family in our life.

The nurse ushered Christopher and me back. I was instructed to remove my clothes and put on the hospital gown, and I did so. Luckily I didn't have to wait long for the doctor, another nurse, and an ultrasound technician to come in. They took my information and chief complaint and covered my bottom half with a blanket. They pulled up my hospital gown and ran the transponder over my belly. I held my breath as they searched for a heartbeat. It was probably seconds, but it felt like hours before strong swishes came on the speakers. The heart was still beating, at least. They rolled the transponder over my belly, taking several pictures and checking every corner until they found the source of the bleeding. A uterine cyst had burst and was bleeding. It was old blood build-up. That was why the blood had been so dark. Everything was still holding strong with our pregnancy, and our baby was healthy. I was so relieved, I choked out a 'thank you' through my tears. He instructed us to come back if the bleeding got worse or started again, but for now, we were in the clear.

We were discharged from the hospital, and after picking up Cayden, we all took a nap in our bed. Miss Nancy and Mr. Dennis volunteered to take Cayden in the afternoon. I was happy they did because by 1:00, I had begun heavily bleeding again, and Christopher and I returned to the emergency room. Once again, they performed an ultrasound and bloodwork. Everything was normal, it was just another cyst, and I needed to be vigilant to watch out for fever or signs of infection with this continuation of bleeding.

We sighed in relief and were once again discharged, and I stayed in bed for the rest of the day. Fighting off flashbacks, snuggling Cayden, Chris, and my dogs.

Last week we received a genetic analysis from the doctor on our new baby. She was healthy! No Osteogenesis, no other looming genetic disorders, and to top it all off, it was a girl. Christopher and I were so happy we cried happy tears. We told our parents with a cute package including a stocking inside and a note that said, "Santa's not the only one coming to town... baby girl due December 21." Both sets of parents reacted cautiously, but were happy for us. They were just concerned about another tragedy, which was understandable, and we were too.

I had called a meeting with Kevin and Richard to report on the pregnancy. They acted happy and congratulated me. The following week, I had my mid-year review. I walked in confidence but dreading it with the dynamic that Richard had engaged with me as of late. I was surprised to see Kevin sitting at the table too, but they explained away that he was there to observe as a new boss.

I sat at the conference table opposite Kevin, and Richard shut the door behind me. There were no windows, and suddenly the room was starting to feel small. He handed me a copy of my review.

Section by section, we reviewed my performance. I had advocated for myself due to the hard work I was doing despite my struggles with my grief, PTSD, and my new pregnancy. He did not feel the same. Every category was a "Does Not Meet," with paragraphs demeaning my efforts and disappointments in my performance. As we approached the end, I was in tears because he shut me down as I rebutted. He shoved a "Performance Improvement Plan" to my side of the table. These plans gave you 90 days to complete tasks to "improve your performance," or you would be fired. Usually, they were basic goals and metrics. This plan was seven pages long, with items I needed to complete by the end of October. I panicked.

How could I do all of this? Hot angry tears fell from my eyes. If they fired me at the end of October, it would mean no short-term disability-maternity leave. No money for food or rent for my family with a new baby. I choked when I tried to talk because I was so distraught. Finally, they dismissed me, and I went to my office and shut the door, balling. How could they do this to me? It wasn't fair. I came back to this place *for them.* Now that I was struggling and pregnant, they were so calloused to jeopardize my family and me?

When I talked to Brian, who was my co-worker in the same district, he confirmed that they had given him a great review and was shocked to find out what they did to me. He told me that I ran the ship and kept everyone together. If they did that to me, what does that say that they would do to the rest of them?

I did not go gently into despair. When I gathered myself, I lined out all of the seven pages of tasks into a timeline with checkpoints. I wrote Candor about how fucking awful and unfair it was and accidentally sent it to Richard. I panicked but was too far gone in my hurt to care. I still had my job after that, so I let it roll off of me.

I fought tooth and nail for three months to reach the checkpoints, the new level of stress in combination with my pregnancy and still being a mom and wife wiped me out and flared my flashbacks. Brian resigned because of the working conditions. It was hell, and I looked forward to Alicia's wedding. I asked them a month earlier to let me know if I still had a job before I left for her wedding in Milwaukee so, at eight months pregnant, I could relax a little.

They didn't, of course. Instead, they harassed me to get a membership. There were hurdles for me to jump through to get a club up and running, and they made me jump through every single one on my train journey to Milwaukee. When I finally got WiFi, I sent the membership package in with help from Rhian and Barb! I did it! I had year-end growth, and the council hit its benchmark. Yes, I was supposed to be off. No, I did not have a choice. I resolved to contact all my leaders to pick up their popcorn for the following Friday on Monday and put my phone on vibrate for the weekend. I was hostess for her Harry Potter-themed-bachelorette, after all!

In true best friend fashion, on Sunday, Alicia and her mom threw me a baby shower with my Chicagoland friends. I was touched by the love and support I was receiving (especially since we were approaching Alicia's big day). As we drove the small jog from Milwaukee to Chicago, Richard called me twice. Alicia and I made eye contact. She was all too familiar with my work situation and what I had endured on Friday. "Do I need to take your phone?" she asked with concern. I told her I knew and put it in my pocket. I was supposed to be off. It was a Sunday. Nothing he said was more important than what I was doing right now, getting ready to be showered with love by people I hadn't seen in *years*. Richard called again, and then my mom called. Richard had called her about popcorn because she was going to help me contact everyone to get their popcorn, but we hadn't started because it was in a week, and she told him as much. He was very rude and angry to her on the phone, for which I apologized to my mom. I texted Richard that I was at my baby shower and I would call him after. He called me four more times during the shower. He then sent me a six-part text message about how irresponsible I was and how I had not lined everyone up to get their popcorn. I simply texted back, "That's because I had to chase down membership paperwork all day on Friday while I was supposed to be off and was on the train. I did not have enough time to contact everyone to schedule it and intended to do it Monday." He asked why I hadn't just told him that. He got me there. I told him that I didn't believe it was an emergency and that I wanted to celebrate my baby shower in peace on my day off.

I did as I promised, set up all of the pick-ups, and rested my very swollen pregnant self while Alicia went to her aerial workout and ran around with her friend from Amsterdam. I spent the week being loved on, cared for, and resting (and intermittently working), and enjoyed Alicia's wedding to Nate.

When I came into work on Monday, tension flared in the office. Kevin and Richard called me into the conference room once more. Richard gritted his teeth, "I am happy to say you beat the work plan. You still have work to do, but you did it. You can sign it here." My relief was clipped short as he slapped another piece of paper down. "However, because of your insubordination, while you were gone, you are being written up. This is a written warning that if anything like that happens again, you will be immediately terminated." "But it was a Sunday, on my days off, and I was at *my* baby shower." "That doesn't matter. You should have lined up those pick-up times weeks ago, and you didn't, and you made me chase down your mother and Ashley to get answers. Sign the document, or you will be let go right now." Hot tears streaked my cheeks in my shock. I signed it and waited until I was dismissed before I walked into my office and cried. If the walls of that office could talk, I would be screwed.

———⬤———

The next month flew by. My sisters-in-law threw me a baby shower. It was perfect and supportive in every way, and I was so thankful. Ember wouldn't have to wear an outfit twice with all of the adorable baby girl clothes we got. Then came time for our final district meeting before my maternity leave began. I prepared for the long day ahead as usual. But I had been working my tail off on nights and weekends to prepare for my leave so the volunteers and youth would be able to go on with business as usual in my absence. I met with Kevin, gave him a detailed plan, and updated him on all parts of my territory.

One of my volunteers, Ella, came in early, and when I told her that I needed to go set up, she said that Rick and Mike were setting up and I didn't have to worry. Barb shut my door for me, and I was suspicious. Ella and I continued to talk about the baby that could come any day but was scheduled for a C-section next Thursday. She and her daughters and grandchildren had been so sweet and helpful even when we went camping at the fall camporee. Yes, at seven months pregnant, I hauled myself out to camp. Luckily Scouts are courteous and kind. I didn't have to hardly lift a finger. They even set up my tent and blew up my air mattress for me, and fed me meals.

The volunteers and their Scouts were like family to me, so when Amber led me to the large conference room, with my eyes covered, I was crying happy tears for the beautiful, camp-themed baby shower they threw for me. They gave us wonderful gifts and talked. Rick and Barb had arranged the whole thing without me having a clue. Hard to do when I felt like I usually knew what was going on in my territory. I thanked each one of them, and they thanked me for all of my hard work and reassured me that they would take care of the district while I was on leave.

CHAPTER 12

I woke up in the middle of the night feeling like I had peed on myself. I picked up my phone. The clock read 12:01 AM. Knowing this pregnancy, it was incredibly possible I peed on myself, but it felt different. I padded to the bathroom around the fluffy dogs. I peed and finished, but fluid still fell from me. Uh-oh. Our C-section wasn't for two more days, and the doctor had made no "plan b" with us about what we should do if I went into labor. We were two weeks before our due date, after all. A massive wave of pain washed over my body from my core and rippled down to my toes. Yes, that was a contraction, and yes, this was it. I stood and pulled up my pants and emerged from the bathroom.

"Chris," I whispered loudly but no stirring, so I just repeated his name out loud. He stirred with a, "What?" "I went to the bathroom, and some fluid came out." "How much?" "A little bit." There was a long pause, and then I heard snoring.

"Christopher!" "What? What!" "Chris, my water broke. We need to go to the hospital. Get up." After a brief groan, he got up. I told him I was going to take a shower since I wouldn't be able to do so for a couple of days. (At least not an enjoyable one, as I had learned from my previous C-section.).

I climbed into the shower. Another contraction flushed over my body, and I braced my arm against the shower wall. I let the waterfall over me, head tilted back, inhaling and exhaling slowly.

A flashback crept up my spine—the final night being pregnant with Hope took over when I had showered like I am now to relax my nerves. My efforts were in vain. As I felt her roll lightly beneath my skin, I wept into the water, knowing these moments would soon be over. That our daughter would be gone tomorrow. Crippling fear pulsed through my veins. *'Our daughter will be gone,'* rang in my ears.

I reached and shut off the water, ripping back the shower curtain to meet the humid air. My eyes fought to focus on the present moment, unstable as my brain focused on the flashback. I made my way over to the sink and splashed my face with cold water, and gasped as I repeated over and over until the flashback ceased.

I looked up at my face, a white sheet. I had to stay at this moment. We would meet our Ember later that day. Hope was gone, but she will always be with us. Today was Ember's day. Another contraction. Yes, I am still in my body,

I put some clothes and some basics into a suitcase for myself. Luckily I had already packed Ember's clothes and boppy, and I really had expected to have two more days to pack and get ready. Our doctor hadn't even checked me periodically like I had been checked with Cayden because he had been so confident that having the C-section a week early would be enough time that I wouldn't go into labor. After all, I had to be induced almost a week late with Cayden and still had to have a C-section.

Chris had been calling Nancy and Dennis with no luck on an answer. I called my co-workers, Barb and Amber. No answer. I called Ashley and Marti, and no answer. This was not good. There was no way Cayden would be allowed to be in the surgery room with us—nor would I want him to be. The boy had been in enough trauma with Hope, and he didn't need to add having his mom be eviscerated to the list. Chris readied his school backpack with extra clothes and his tablet, and a very sleepy Cayden strolled into the hallway.

Chris ushered the dogs into their kennels as I continued to try Nancy and Dennis. They must have their ringers off, and why would they have them on? Ember wasn't supposed to be here for two more days! When he returned, we exited the house, stepping into the cool, crisp air. The cold was a relief on my body that had strained with a few more leg-crippling contractions before we had left the house. She was undoubtedly coming on strong.

The drive to the hospital was a short five minutes, but I swear I called Nancy 5 more times before we got there. Luckily we had at least visited the hospital, so we knew where to go. It was 1:00 AM by then, so we went to the emergency room. I was still having contractions and felt the warm fluid continue to come with each one. The triage nurse took my vitals, and then they whisked the three of us into a room to do hospital paperwork because I had just completed it and turned it in this afternoon, and it hadn't made it into the system yet. Naturally, as is our luck, I had to fill out all of the forms *again*, deep breathing, contractions and all. Chris tried to help as much as he could, but to be honest, the talking was infuriating me while I was trying to focus more than anything. Somehow I had to get these forms filled out, stay in the moment, and breathe through the labor, while battling off flashbacks that I could feel like a cold fluid in my mind and trickling down my back. Yes, it was a big fucking mess.

When I finally completed the forms, Chris had still not gotten through to Nancy and Dennis. It was finally time for them to wheel me up to the maternity ward. The three of us, plus a nurse who was pushing the wheelchair, went on the long walk upstairs. They found us a large delivery suite that we would only briefly get to enjoy. Labor was starting to set in earnest now, and with it, flashbacks crept along, briefly popping up. Images of our day with Hope wrenching their way into my line of sight, my heart pounding as my mind tried to sort out the mess. I had been off of my flashback medication since we found out we were pregnant, and now the chief stimulus that kept me present in my own body was the contractions. I wasn't ready to go through this. I still needed those two more days to mentally prepare. Tears welled in my eyes as the terror set in. Christopher instructed Cayden to turn around as I changed into two hospital gowns. One to cover the front side and one to cover my backside. A few nurses came into the room and strapped itchy monitors to my belly. Ember kept rolling away from the monitors, so trying to catch her heart rate was a moving target.

A maternity nurse introduced herself to me as Theresa. She had come to check me and test the fluid to make sure that it was amniotic fluid. As she uncovered me and Chris stepped in front of Cayden to break his line of sight, a large contraction rippled over me. "Wait," I wheezed. I didn't want anything near me down there while I was trying to breathe through this. When it ceased, the nurse said, "Wow! That was a big one. I am going to check you and do the test now." I am sure she had perfectly delicate hands, but it felt like her whole fucking fist went up there, and the test felt sharp against my sore cervix. I am sure she heard me gasp as a flash of the small room from Hope's day flickered in and out of focus.

I announced that I had to pee so I could cry in the bathroom. I was ashamed that the flashbacks were ruining this time with Ember, but I couldn't stop it. This was the day that I was scared of. The setting and circumstances were too familiar.

I held onto the bar next to the toilet as the flashbacks ran rampant in my mind. Tears streaming down my face, cold sweat beading on my temple as I let myself fall apart for a moment because I needed to. This should have been my labor with Hope, and I grieved that fact in private.

When I washed my hands and emerged from the bathroom, I felt all worried eyes on me. I reminded myself that Ember and I were the stars of the show today and brushed it off. I returned to the bed, and Theresa informed me that they had alerted the doctor and he would be on his way soon. Christopher was going to take Cayden to Nancy and Dennis' house since they still didn't answer. He would just bang on the door, and hopefully, the dogs would wake them up. I gave him a hug and a kiss and gave Cayden a firm hug and a big kiss and told him I loved him. Anxiety from my grandmother's surgery that led to her death always loomed with large medical events for me. He took Cayden out of the room, so it was just the nurse and me. I asked her if my doctor would be doing the surgery. Unfortunately, she told me that not him but the OB/GYN partner from his practice would be standing in—Dr. Prendergast.

The doctor was a board member of the non-profit I worked for. He was kind and friendly, and if he wasn't a board member, I would have asked him to be my doctor from the beginning because, to be honest, how awkward was it going to be for him to look me in the eye after seeing ALL of ME at my most vulnerable. But, here we are, 3:00 AM, 2 days earlier than my scheduled C-section, and he was doing the surgery. "Just don't expect him to be his cheery self. He seemed pretty cranky on the phone. We just didn't want you to suffer more than you have to if you are going to end up with a C-section anyway," Nurse Theresa explained.

It seemed like no time had passed when they started preparing me for surgery. Spiking my IV bag, getting me standing. I panicked. Chris wasn't back yet, there was no way in hell I was doing this without him, and I told the nurses as much. So we waited, and right before the final call for me to go down the hall to the surgery suite, he came through the door. He wiggled on the scrubs and hair cap over his clothes; being a 6'5" man meant that standard scrubs simply did not cover all of him. He took my hand, and we walked quietly down the hallway with the nurse and my IV bag trailing alongside. He kissed my hand and smiled, "We're having a baby today." I smiled back, "We're having a baby today." We stepped into the surgical suite.

It was abuzz with activity. Nurses and medical students were here, there, and everywhere preparing. The doctor had just arrived at the hospital, and they were going to have the anesthesiologist put in a spinal block while we waited for the doctor to prep. The anesthesiologist was a short, squat man who constantly mumbled. He managed to clearly instruct me to remove my back hospital gown and wipe my back down with iodine. This part hurt like a son of a bitch with Cayden. My muscles started to tighten and ripple up my back, becoming a solid brick wall. He managed to clearly tell me not to move. Christopher and Theresa stood in front of me and held my hands. I felt one needle burn like a branding iron as it went in. I cried out, and BAM!

The veil fell between me and everyone around me. I was in that small dark room, and Hope was being pulled apart in pieces. Her feet were pressed to the page with ink, one leg separated from her body. I surfaced briefly as the anesthesiologist removed the catheter and stuck me AGAIN and AGAIN, digging in my back. I panted and struggled against the flashbacks. Christopher recognized it and tried to keep my eye contact, "It's not real. You are here with us. It's not real." He held onto me tight until the doctor finally placed the needle in my back accurately. Finally, the numbness began to spread in my legs and travel up my waist. The nurses quickly moved to my side to help me place my legs on the table and laid my back down gently. I started to panic. I was scared of the surgery, scared for my baby but also for myself.

The anesthesiologist took care of that. He spiked me with something and placed an oxygen tube in my nose. I started to relax, and the flashbacks began to die down as Dr. Prendergast entered the room. He came up to my head to say hi and let me know he was going to take good care of us today. His eyes were kind, and I could tell that even if he was tired and cranky, he was smiling behind his medical mask. They erected the sheet to separate my head and chest from the rest of my body so I wouldn't see my insides on the outside and go into shock. So long as everything was okay with Ember, they let me have skin-to-skin contact with her while they closed me up, which made me happy.

I should have known better.

It seemed like no time, and several big pulls later, that Dr. Prendergast hollered, "Stand up, dad!" Christopher stood and watched the doctor pull Ember from the incision in my belly. He held her up over the sheet for me, and she let out a very polite little cry. My heart filled with love at the very first sight of her. That little cry was one of the only sounds she made. They called Chris over for pictures and to watch over her, but I didn't hear anything besides murmurs behind me, and I couldn't turn my head around to see what was happening. Yes, I agreed with myself. It was far too quiet. I felt the drowsy, anti-anxiety medication start to drag my senses. "What's going on? Where's my baby," I managed. Dr. Prendergast came around the sheet and explained that Ember wasn't breathing as well as they would like, and they were going to take her to the NICU to get her some help. Panic struck me in a deep maternal way. Christopher came up by my side and held my head. I could tell he was conflicted as on one end, his wife was still eviscerated on a surgical table, and in the other room was his daughter, fighting for her life. "Go," I instructed him, "Go take care of our baby. I'm fine. There is nothing I can do. Just go be with

Ember." He asked me if I was sure, to which I told him absolutely, and he rushed out of the room, following the medical team that had Ember in tow.

The doctors and nurses told me to rest and to just go to sleep while they closed me up. Fat. Fucking. Chance. I willed myself against the drug haze. I had to stay conscious. I had to know what was happening to my baby. I had already surrendered to the medication over a year ago, and all it did was leave me deeply scarred. I would stay awake, albeit loopy, but awake and expect updates on our daughter.

They finally closed me up and moved me into recovery, where Chris rejoined me. He said that Ember was stable and breathing with the help of a C-Pap, and she would be okay, but it was pretty much touch-and-go for a second. He told me her color looked much better than when she was in the delivery room. The doctors said it sometimes happens with C-section babies because they don't get the final 'squeeze' and big inhale like naturally born babies that's why, sometimes they just don't breathe initially. I asked the nurse when I could go see our daughter. She told me when my vitals came back up and I recovered for a little while, I could go see her.

I don't know how to describe the urgency. I felt like a wounded animal with its young on the other side of a ravine. It was primal. I wanted to see and hold my baby. I waited impatiently as the blood pressure cuff took and retook my blood pressure automatically. I asked Chris to text my dad and let him know what was going on along with Michon and Nancy. Chris told me that Nancy had been texting since they got Cayden. I asked him to go back and be with our daughter. I was okay and just wanted him to be with her in case something changed. He gave me a kiss and reluctantly left the room. He left me with my phone, and I texted people back, letting some others know that Ember was here, but pictures would have to follow later.

I was scared, even with the medication making me groggy. At last, the nurse said I could move into my maternal suite. First, they set me all the way up and took me to see Ember on the gurney. I didn't get to hold her yet because I was still groggy. What frightened me were all of the lines coming off of her. A feeding tube, IV and heart monitor leads and a pulse ox were attached to her, but it wasn't as alarming as the C-pap machine that covered most of her little face. Through all of that, I could tell how beautiful she was. My heart that had set dark and dormant like a dead star burned again in my chest, warming my soul with love for our new daughter. I held her little hand, and she gripped my index finger in response. It was hard to turn over to her, but I managed.

After a while, the nurses told me that we all needed rest, so Christopher headed home to shower and take a nap, and they wheeled my gurney into my hospital room. I had my own room and bathroom, which I would share with Ember when she was strong enough.

Several nurses came in, gripped the sheet beneath me, and helped lift me onto the hospital bed. I cried out, and it felt like I was being pulled in half. Not to be alarmed, though. This was actually a normal feeling for C-section patients, or at least was how I felt when I had Cayden. I was extremely sleepy, but the pain shot through me like lightning, and I began to shiver, my teeth chattering. The nurses were kind and gave me an extra blanket, before they dimmed the lights so I could take a nap. When I woke up, I could go see my baby again. I was overwhelmed with love and gratitude and finally closed my eyes to rest.

No rest came. Just as I was starting to drift off, sharp pains started in my abdomen. That was new for me, so I called the nurse, and she came quickly. When I told her what was happening, she smiled and replied, "I guess you aren't going to get that nap after all. That is the gas pain you are feeling. We have to get you up and moving to make it go away. Do you want to try walking to the NICU? We will follow you with a wheelchair, and whenever you get tired, we can roll you the rest of the way." I was excited at the thought of seeing my daughter again, so when the nurse helped me sit up and move my legs to the side of the bed, I used all my energy to do so. I wanted to be with my new baby—it was my basic instinct. I held onto my IV pole and my catheter bag (classy, I know) as the nurses draped a second gown around my backside like a cape to cover up my back-end. I immediately felt unstable on my own two feet and used a pillow at my incision to hold my guts in, hunched over when my legs shook as I walked. I willed myself to walk down that hall to see my baby. I made it about halfway before my legs shook so hard that my knees actually knocked. The nurses were right behind me and in front of me with a wheelchair in tow, so when I wore down, I was able to sit quickly. They wheeled me the rest of the way to the NICU as promised, and I got to see Ember.

Ember was stable enough now that they actually let me hold her. I nuzzled her as she curled up into me. I couldn't nurse her yet with the C-pap, but I didn't care. I was just so thankful she was here. She was safe. Tears of joy came but so did the tears of grief. I longed to be able to hold our Hope this way. That is the funny thing about grief. From the moment you lose someone that critical in your life, all of your happiest moments will always be a little sad because they aren't there with you.

I held her on and off all day, especially when I was finally able to feed her. What was absolutely precious was when Chris brought Cayden to meet his baby sister in the NICU. I held her bundled in my arms, and Cayden stroked her head and kept repeating, "My baby sister." He glowed with pride and watched her dutifully, and, like she had been waiting for him, she opened her eyes for the first time and smiled. Even when we put her back in the bassinet to have her diaper changed, Cayden stood by and gave her the binky that had rolled out of her mouth (it was only onto the bassinet, not the floor). Miss Nancy sent flowers and came to visit and held Ember with the pride of a new grandmother. My mother came from Manhattan to check on me, and other volunteers came to visit, which was more than I could have hoped for.

It was a happy moment when Ember was able to break out of the NICU. It was a beautiful, earth-shattering moment when Cayden gingerly sat in my lap, and Christopher handed Cayden his baby sister. Cayden gave her kisses and nuzzled her, and she cooed back. My heart swelled with love for our little family, one more member richer.

That night, in between feedings with Ember in the bassinet, I talked to Hope. I told her how I wished she were here, and she would forever be my baby. I told her that while Ember was here on earth, she did not replace her but my heart had grown to fit all of them, and I hoped she would understand.

CHAPTER 13

When my maternity leave ended, I did not want to go back to work. Richard was gone and had been promoted, but Kevin still remained, and I didn't trust men who had two volumes: silent or yelling. I returned to a hostile environment. The new boss they had brought in to replace Richard, Pete, was nice enough, but so much damage had been done. He was kind and upbeat, and candid, which I appreciated.

It just wasn't the same—my passion for the Boy Scouts had been beaten out of me. I tried, but the depth of the betrayal that I felt from when I was pregnant with Ember and mourning Hope ran deep. For eight years, my vision for myself had been to work full-time and be in charge at Philmont. But I could feel my purpose, my vision for myself crumbling beneath me.

In addition to having an identity crisis with my career, my marriage was rocky at best. We had been trying couples therapy but were failing, and I stopped going to therapy altogether. I also stopped getting my prescriptions refilled. I had begun to lash out, shaking and scared from the raging flashbacks. I felt like a useless mother and sobbed for feeling like I was not honoring Hope. I fought with Christopher but, in the same breath, mourned our friendship.

I was unstable, and one night I couldn't take it anymore. I wrote letters to my family, words of closure that it wasn't their fault, and I made a plan to end my life. I would park the car on the side of I70, and I walk in front of a semi-truck. It would be over fast. No more flashbacks, no more need for a purpose. I could finally rest.

The next morning Christopher noticed I was acting weird, and as he did before, he forced me to see Allison. It took some prying, but Allison drew my plan out of me, as well as the fact that I had been off my medication and not in therapy with anyone else. She reckoned that I needed to be inpatient immediately. She called Christopher to come and get me to take me to the hospital. He was angry at me for being selfish enough to want to kill myself. He waited with me in the emergency room in silence until he had to pick Cayden up from school. After that, I was on my own.

The stay at the hospital was 72 hours. Chris brought the kids to see me once. We just told them and my bosses that I was sick— I was sick... just in my mind. They stabilized my mood with medications and forced me to do heavy introspection. I was released on the condition that I followed up with my medications and restarted psychotherapy. I agreed to both. It was the hard reset that I needed.

I began to cling to the idea of being a non-profit CEO so that I could make sure that anyone that I took charge of never felt this way. I believed the missions to be true norths for non-profits, and I was determined to find one where I could exercise my CEO prowess. This new sense of purpose pulled me forward and gave me the strength to leave the Boy Scouts of America.

ADVOCATE
[PART 4]

When I left the hospital after my breakdown, I vowed to get out of the Boy Scouts and leave the toxicity behind me for good. I felt terrible for leaving Pete, he had been really kind to me, but I knew I would end up back in the hospital if I stayed. I interviewed a few places before my friend Marti connected me with the YMCA. She told me to apply for a membership position I was wildly overqualified for, but it would get me out of the job I was currently in. Angie, the president, and CEO had been best friends with my old boss Wendy before she left for Texas, so when she saw my name roll across her desk (or rather Marti marched in her office to tell her that she should hire me… thank you, Marti!), she called me in for a meeting. When I sat across from her in her office, the first words, she said, "Okay, you have my attention. I am curious why you are applying to work at the front desk. You've always been such a huge advocate for the Boy Scouts. What's going on?" I told her in the most tactful way I could that the culture had turned increasingly toxic since Wendy had left and that I was burned out and needed a change. My mission was to become a non-profit CEO one day, and I thought I could learn that from the YMCA.

Unfortunately, at the time, she did not have a position open for me that would fulfill me in the way that I was seeking, but the door was open if things got really bad so that I could come work at the front desk. I thanked her for her time and consideration and left, feeling a little deflated. It felt like I was trying to catch a cloud while pursuing this new dream of mine.

A week or two passed, and Angie called me back. Their membership director had moved on, and the position was open, and she wanted to interview me for the position in combination with my fundraising talents. After two rounds of interviews, I became her new Director of Member and Donor Relations. I was thrilled to be able to focus on the big picture work and manage my own teams. I would be able to start working towards my goal and step into a true leadership role with a title I had earned.

Before I even started my job at the Salina Family YMCA, I came in to turn in the paperwork to get started a few weeks later, I was sitting with Angie. I had noticed a particular line in the dress code notes, so I asked, "Angie, I know that in the dress code it remarks that all tattoos must be covered, but I have a pair of footprints from my baby that passed away on my neck, which will be visible when I put my hair up, and I don't feel comfortable covering them." I held my breath. I was coming from a very toxic work environment, and I needed this job to be set free.

"I'm glad you said something," Angie responded with a warm smile, "I have been meaning to change this line in the dress code to reflect that just vulgar tattoos need to be covered. I have a tattoo on my ankle." I sighed in relief, "Thank you, I was really worried."

On my first day of work, it was stiflingly hot. It was late May in the middle of Kansas after all, and I put my hair up intermittently. Angie must have seen my tattoo then because my hair was down but swept to the side when I returned to my desk. She approached my desk and asked, "Tell me about your baby?" I, of course, thought she was talking about our 5-

month-old daughter Ember, so I simply responded, "She is 5 months old and fiery but at the same time the sweetest baby you will meet." "Yes, I have met Ember, but tell me about your baby whose footprints you have tattooed. You don't have to talk about it if you don't want to but just know I am here to listen." I froze. No one ever asked about Hope, but there she was with a kind smile on her face. I gave her a very abridged version that she had a terrible genetic condition, and we had lost her when we were 18 weeks pregnant. She showed me her ankle tattoo and replied that she had lost a baby too. Her baby Ethan came too soon, and he had passed away after he was born. My eyes met hers with a knowing only moms like us could share. The sharing of hell and grief and love for an angel who was taken too soon from this world.

"I had no idea," I told her, "I have known you for a while and had no idea." I had met Angie several times over the years of being with my previous job, and while she had been closer with my previous boss Wendy, she hadn't even connected the two of us together then. I wondered if Wendy had even known. Angie told me sweetly that was why she had "E" decorations and elephants in her office and her necklace with Ethan's toe prints, to always remind her that Ethan was watching over her.

My heart ached in a familiar way for her, Ethan, and Hope. I asked her if it would ever get any easier, to which she smiled and told me that medicine helps and it changes, but it doesn't really go away. I giggled at the medication comment. I told her that I feel like I am a walking pharmacy sometimes, and she laughed back, "Yes, good meds were a good thing. I still takes the good meds."

Angie brought me so much hope and inspiration that day. She was a woman who was where I wanted to be, a CEO of a non-profit—and carried the grief of the loss of a child with so much love in her heart. She met life and being a manager with so much compassion and empathy that it gave me a little spark for myself.

A little Hope.

Angie and I had spent a long session in her craft room assembling the 50th-anniversary cake topper for my mother and father-in-law. It was a beast to tackle because of the glitter cardstock. We had talked about everything from work to Hope to family dynamics. She asked if we would attend her Super Bowl party, to which I responded, "Of course." Chris was going to be a wreck as the Chiefs were playing for the first time in fifty years, but I needed some help from other adults to run interference with the kiddos so that they wouldn't bother him as much while he was locked in on the game.

On Super Bowl day, I made chicken enchilada dip and some lemon bars—two of his favorites and made some Rotel/Velveeta dip he loved, trying to make the party experience as positive of one as I could. When we arrived at Angie's house, she slipped a small white box into my hand. She told me it was a mom box for me when I was having a moment and to not open it until I was in a quiet place. I agreed and placed it in the diaper bag to come home. We watched the game, Ember snuggled Angie, and Todd and Cayden played with them. Overall it was a good night.

We returned home, and the Chiefs just pulled off the win. After our kiddos went to bed, I pulled out the box and opened it. I understood why she told me to open it when I have a quiet space. It was a box made for the mother of an Angel. The first piece of content was a wooden Hope ornament from Angie's Christmas tree. I knew it was from her tree because I remember seeing it adorning her tree a couple of months earlier. I kissed it and held it to my chest, and then set it aside. I pulled out another ornament. This one had tiny foam balls like snow inside and read, "Snowflakes are just kisses from heaven." My heart warmed at the thought. Finally, I pulled out a cross? No, a bird? I wasn't sure. It was made from wood from the YMCA in Israel, though I knew how special it was. This box was for the bad days, to help ground me in memory of Hope. Maybe she had a box like this herself for Ethan. This was a great kindness that I was thankful for.

⸺◦⸺

The pandemic rocked the world in 2020. For Christopher and me, it was a transformative time in our marriage. We began to re-evaluate our priorities, and two things rang out loud—we needed to start putting our family and our marriage first. My grandfather was getting older, and so were his parents. Time with them was precious more than ever, and we both had felt guilty for spending the last several years at a distance, especially after my grandfather's heart attack and fall in 2018. We made the decision to move to Kansas City in June, making the start of the next school year the goal to be moved by. Angie was understanding. The pandemic made so many re-evaluate their values and priorities.

There were a lot of starts and stops, but by the end of August, we were moved into Christopher's parents' house for two months before settling into our own home with our own jobs and childcare. I began leadership coaching with Amanda, a previous President of the United Way who began her coaching business right before the pandemic hit. I had always respected and admired her, and I was excited to learn from her. Our first order of business was to set goals for our time together. They included:

1. Establish a direction for my career path

2. Establish my core values and rediscover my strengths

3. Write a book about my experiences

If you are reading this, you know I have accomplished at least
one of these.

CHAPTER 15

It is amazing what can trigger you. It is obnoxious that "triggering" or "trigger words" or being "triggered" is a joke now. A pop culture reference that was warped from what is a symptom of a debilitating disease. Let me tell you what being triggered is really like.

Put a gun to your head.

Pull the trigger.

Not literally, of course, but for the purpose of this practice, visualize it. Let's pretend for this exercise that it is an old-school, western-style gun with a six-pocket chamber. When a traumatic event occurs, it fills these chambers with bullets. As the traumatic event closes, it snaps the gun shut when the body exits the heightened adrenaline state. You spin the chamber closed, pull the hammer back and wait, with your finger still on the trigger.

Only, it's not really you with your finger on the trigger. Hell, it's not even really you holding the gun. It is your post-traumatic stress disorder. You see, when the gun snapped shut, the traumatic event manifested a heavy unworldly being—a dark force that envelopes you, filling your veins with cement as it places its neurons on top of yours. A symbiote that folds itself around you, with its finger is on the trigger of the gun, holding it to your head.

Anything can cause the trigger finger to squeeze and set off the gun. A smell, a taste, a sound, a song: anything. Somewhere your PTSD symbiote has stuck a connection between the trauma and the stimuli. That connection acts like a hook embedded into the trigger finger, attached to a line; like a puppet master, the symbiote pulls on that string, and the finger squeezes, setting off the gun in response to the stimuli. The bullet causes a catastrophic cascade of a veil that separates me from the rest of the world—on the veil replays horrors from that week. Some are repetitive. Others are new, pieces of my memory coming back from the midazolam. The result is a crippling, frozen state while the sensory overload takes over in a flashback. I am detached from reality. The only past, present, and future is now, in this moment of terror.

People ask why I still have flashbacks. Do I ever think they will go away? Don't I take medicine for it?

The truth is I have lived a life full of violence, physical, mental, and sexual abuse. Each one was putting another bullet in the chamber. What happened to Hope just filled it up and snapped the chamber shut, and kept the hammer pulled back. The medicine helps take the bullets from the chamber, but there is always a possibility that this trigger will fire a bullet, or sometimes, a blank. At least with a bullet, I know what to expect. A blank makes a loud noise still but can be unpredictable. It still causes a physical response and demands a quick acknowledgment of the memory. Sometimes I get lucky. The medicine does its job, and while the trigger clicks, there is no bullet to echo and cause cascading systems failure. The longer and more consistent I stay on my meds, the more empty the chamber. I had the pleasantry of having a couple of no fires, a couple of blanks and bullets the weekend we visited friends on a trip to Saint Louis.

No Fire

Our friends were trying to have a baby. The only baby we ever tried for was Hope. The trigger squeezed. Click. Nothing. No shot from the barrel. I could move on with my day.

We watch a grueling horror film. Zombies are attacking everywhere. Gore everywhere. It isn't until the pregnant zombie queen is beheaded and the king rips open her abdomen that Chris tells me to quickly close my eyes and I looked away fixating my gaze on his face as our friend fast forwarded until we are well past the scene. The trigger was squeezed harder this time. Click. Nothing. I was lucky that time.

Blank

It was the following morning. We joked about 'fancy' and 'classy' date spots, and our friend joked about Red Lobster. The trigger clicked, and BANG! A blank exploded inside my head. I wondered if the same thing was happening in my husband's head, too, because before I was able to put words into my thoughts, he responded, "I don't think we have visited Red Lobster since Hope died." "Yeah," I echoed, "We wanted a crab melt before…" "Before our life fell apart," he finished. That was the first time I felt like we experienced even a part of Hope's death together. Like I wasn't forcing my grief onto him. Letting it out, talking about it was so new and so foreign to me. Understanding that was not something normal and for the first time in years, I felt a spark, just a flicker of our love for each other return. It was so loving and organic to recognize the blank together that I did not feel alone for the first time in four years.

My son was overjoyed to receive Beyblades for his eighth birthday. They are little tops that wound with a ripcord on a handle. "Wound" is too gentle of a phrase, and CRANK is more accurate. The CRANK and the ripcord are made of hard plastic, so it makes a heavy squeaking sound when wound. Over and over.

BAM!

A blank fire in my head. We didn't know what would happen to Hope's body on our way to and from the procedure, so we brought a foam cooler in the car. Just in case a funeral home refused to pick up her body, we would bring it to Manhattan, where my mom arranged a funeral home to take her, but we would have to transport her to Manhattan. What we didn't realize was how the squeaking of the foam at every road bump would become a capstone scar in our brains. *The squeak. The squeak.*

The squeak.

A squeak like the plastic on our son's toy. I breathed in and breathed out and felt my fists tighten and close on my leggings, my jaw clenching. It was his new favorite toy, so I waited, locked up, doing my best to keep it together. Grounding myself to keep a flashback at bay, but I felt it creeping in. Finally, I asked Cayden for just five more 'rips'. He agreed to my terms, and after five more ranks, he played with a different toy.

It was finally over. I softened my jaw, unclenched my fingers, and rubbed my sore, white knuckles. My breathing slowed down, and the mist that was starting to cloud my mind dissipated.

Bullet

We were all exhausted and hot, but our trip to the Saint Louis Zoo had been a beautiful family time with our littles and our Philmont Friends. We piled into the minivan we rented and began our drive to the house. The radio DJ announced that

Mike Shenandoah did a collaboration for the next song. Mike Shenandoah, I thought. I guess he needed something to do since Linkin Park lost Chester. Lost Chester. Mike Shenandoah. Chester is dead. There is no more Linkin Park. There is no more Chester. There is no more Hope. The gun fired, and our reality melted away.

No, really. It melts.

The ceiling of the van poured in like lava, and the veil dropped. I heard four-year-old Cayden singing "the light song," which is "One More Light" by Linkin Park. A song he and I clung to when hope died. Their lead singer had died barely a month before Hope, and it was one of the last songs the band had released. I grabbed the seat of the car, trying to ground myself in desperation. I heard my voice screaming for life, for death somewhere distant. I started to rock, trying to ground, trying to snap out of it.

My mind raged. I was crying and holding Cayden. My second worst horror was my inability to protect him from his grief. He crumbled, and I was alone again. I was begging the funeral director to just pick up my baby, who had been lying in a box somewhere for three days. "Please, just get my baby. Please, her name is Hope, and we love her. Please just get my baby," I begged—helpless and guilty for leaving her in Kansas City. I didn't know what to do in Salina, Kansas.

Suddenly, my world started shaking, I felt the yanking of my leg, and I felt myself dropping. No. There was pressure on my leg. I struggled to focus. It was my husband's hand lightly rubbing the inside of my calf and my ankle. I zeroed in on that sensation, and finally, I grounded. I closed my eyes, and I was back in the minivan. The structure was intact, and everyone was unaware of my trip to hell.

———⊶⊶———

In April of 2021, I began working for a non-profit with an Executive Director who deeply valued mental health. She valued mental health so much that the company paid for the employees to go to therapy. It was a godsend for me. I had been without psychotherapy for several months while we were getting established in Kansas City. I started therapy with Chelsea by Zoom with the intention that we would transition to

Eye Movement Desensitization Processing (EMDR). It was easy to do from work, and Chelsea was sweet and didn't shy away when I unloaded the cliff notes of all of my trauma in the first session. I respected her for that. We built up our trust for a few months before it was time to try EMDR.

I was not prepared for that first session. The timeline of EMDR was to start with the trauma that was the most invasive in your life, then go back to the beginning of your trauma and work your way forward. Yep, you Tarantino, your trauma. For me, that was the trauma surrounding Hope. She had me get comfortable on the couch and pick out something that grounded me. I flinched at the thought of the plush blanket, remembering the red plush blanket from that day. She held out a cube box full of different fidgets. I picked out a small wire spring ring. It was slightly pokey and could easily roll between my fingers, and I affectionately named it "pokey."

I settled into the couch, and she had me close my eyes. She had me picture a space where all of my biggest supporters were. For me, it was my old high school football stadium on the aluminum bleachers. One by one, she had me introduce them. My Grams, Christopher, Jamie, Alicia, Sandy, and Miss Nancy, were sitting in a circle on the bleachers. She had me thank them for coming to support me, tell them that I was going on this journey of hard work, tell them to stay there, and I would come back to them. She asked me what they said to me. I could hear my Grams say as clear as day in my ear, *"Keep going."* A shiver rolled up my spine.

She then had me picture a room. Not one I had been in before, an imaginary room, and at the center was a large table with chairs surrounding it. A yellow room came into my vision with a high-top dark wooden table. A single pendant light dimly illuminated the room. She then told me to invite all of the parts of me to sit at the table. I sat at the head of the table, and one by one, parts of me walked into the room. First, a tired mom and wife, Kelsey, came into the room. Her shirt was stained, eyes baggy, and hair in a top knot. Next came Philmont Kelsey. With a bounce in her step, she brightened the room with her spirit. Then came boss-babe Kelsey, commanding the room and giving directions. Next came rebellious, justice-seeking Kelsey. The last one to arrive entered without a sound. The "sad one" with dark black circles around her eyes, which were sunken in her cheeks, tattered clothes, and wind-whipped hair arrived at my left side and placed her hand on my arm. She was the one I had left at the bottom of the storm four years ago. She had returned, silent and with knowing eyes.

Chelsea then had me thank them all for coming and tell them we were about to go on that journey. Each part of me reacted differently, but the sad one squeezed my arm and simply nodded. The message was clear.

Keep going.

Chelsea had me leave the conference room with the parts of me and go to my happy place. The top of the Tooth of Time, lying there with my back on a boulder. The warmth of the rock and the sun shining kindled my spirit. The cool breeze whispering in my ear and birds flying above. Blue skies with puffy white clouds meandered by. That place was my peace. I was safe there.

She then had me leave that place. She wanted me to picture the worst part of Hope's death. It didn't take long before the visual of her body without a head overtook my vision, and tears immediately streamed down my face. I squeezed pokey in my fingers to ground myself, so I wouldn't slip entirely into a flashback. She then had me open my eyes and had me tell her the details of where I was in the memory. She held up two fingers, telling me to follow them with my eyes, and rapidly moved them back and forth, slowly my brain started to associate other places. We would pause and check-in with "what came up" in my thoughts but repeated the rapid eye movements over and over. Eventually, we recalled the original memory. It was the same memory, but it was less 'loud' to me. I was finally able to associate a word with that moment: powerless.

⟐

My second session of EMDR was more challenging than the first, but it was in my third that I felt a shift inside.

Powerless

I had associated my trauma with being powerless, and I was, at that moment, literally powerless. Chelsea deduced that the feeling went deeper back than just my trauma with Hope, though, and she was right. There had been several traumas in my story that had made me powerless in my past. I picked up Pokey, got comfortable on the couch, and closed my eyes. She had me remember back as early as I could to when I had felt powerless. A memory struck from when I was a child, screaming and fighting to try to get back to my Grams. She had me open my eyes and hold that memory. She held up her two fingers and rapidly moved them back and forth, paused, had me take a deep breath, and explained what came up. We continued to evolve my thoughts until an adult me was interfering in my memory.

I picked up little Kelsey, held her close, and told the force they could not have me. That I was taking me back. Chelsea had me repeat the eye sequence. Suddenly I was screaming, wind whipping my face,

"You can't have me. I'm taking me back! I'm taking me baaaack!"

A smile crept across my face, and my eyes met Chelsea's. I recanted what had happened. She was excited for me and suggested that I wasn't just taking myself back. I was taking

back my power. She was right. I felt it being restored.

I am taking me back.

CHAPTER 16

The last few months have been agonizing with triggers. The Supreme Court is in the news, again debating Roe V. Wade, so the trickle-down happens. Some jackasses in Texas, giving women the death penalty if they have an abortion and then the "heartbeat" bill that the Supreme Court let pass.

People take very hard stances they know nothing about. The line is very hard to draw. Pro-Choice and Pro-Life. Do you want to know what someone thinks that has had one? Can you handle the truth?

First, the names of each side are archaic. Let's start with pro-life. Let me tell you right now to fuck right off if you fall into this category. If you think you will find love from this mama, you have been mistaken. Do not use my book, my mental aftermath, as a testament to your pedestal you sit so highly on. Pro-Life means you are for life. All life? No, don't back away.

Are you pro my life? Are you pro wanting to save my life? Then you understand why I would want to save my life too.

Carrying Hope to term with her broken bones, not knowing what the 'term' length would be, was life-threatening to her and to me.

But you don't actually care about the mother, do you? I chose to have sex without protection, so I deserve the consequences. You got me there. We were having sex without protection, and I was even so bold to say I went to Planned Parenthood to get my IUD removed because, guess what? We were trying to have a baby. I know the mind boggles for me to say that the very baby we wanted, we tried for was the baby that could kill me.

No, Pro-Life doesn't care about the mother's well-being. What about children? That's what you're all about, right, saving the children? What about Cayden's life? What about watching mommy's belly grow and then baby sister arrives dead? What if his mommy dies when he is just four years old? Does he deserve to endure these life-changing traumas? No, the most loving-hearted kid in the world does not deserve it. Those traumas are ones you don't come back from, especially at a young age.

No, I guess Pro-Life does not mean pro his life either. What about my husband's life? He is the one who, for ten days, watched me like a ticking time bomb. Did you want to drag that out for weeks, months? Did you want to strain his love for his family so thin? Did you want him to be a widower if I died and raise Cayden on his own?

I guess that means you aren't pro his life either. Whose life are you for then? That's right. My baby's life. Let me tell you what Hope's life had been up to this point.

Every breath was a rib broken… every kick that I cherished was a bone broken into a 90-degree angle. Every time I walked, moved, or sneezed, it meant a broken bone for my baby. Pain was all she knew. I can only hope and pray she knew we loved her, but we knew for sure that she was in unspeakable pain.

That is the life we would have her sentenced to without her only option. You are pro for her to live this way.

The term Pro-Choice is insulting to me. The fact is we didn't have a *choice*, and it was our only *option*. An option is not the same as a choice. Choice infers that there is an independent decision; a choice is something you make for dinner or let your toddler pick what color cup they want. An indication of joy from making a choice.

There was no joy in our option to terminate our pregnancy. We are thankful that the option was possible. It made it so that we didn't drag our baby's suffering out. We didn't walk on eggshells around my belly to worry about her next broken bones for months. We did what we thought would save my life, even when sometimes I wish I were dead.

So no. I don't like the term Pro-Choice, but Pro-Option should be our term to describe the feeling towards this viewpoint.

For all you Pro-Lifers—the pastor that told me that my baby and I are going to hell, the seven churches that turned me down when I asked you to bless Hope's ashes—there's a special place you can go.

I had been writing this book for months when the decisions in Texas and Mississippi were being made, but it was my outrage at the injustice of these rulings that propelled me forward. The marches for women's reproductive rights were being formed, and I knew I had to do something to get the word out about Hope and My story. I quickly pulled together a domain, a website, and a QR code. I called it all "From The Green Desk" because I literally write on a peacock green desk. I then used my Cricut to make a clean sign. I had a resolve as I designed it. I wanted it to get attention and make people discuss the reality of abortion. The sign read, "Our BABY was SUFFERING & DYING, and I would have DIED. Read the truth. fromthegreendesk.com."

I made a t-shirt and a sweatshirt in my signature green with "From The Green Desk" in gold and made flyers and stickers with the QR code. I wanted anyone who would listen to hear about what had happened to Hope and me. My coworker even braided back one side of my hair so that Hope's feet were visible.

When I woke up the morning of the march, anxiety crept in. I was scared because my sign was so personal and significant, and I would be walking this march alone. Cayden had a football game, and while Chris completely supported me in my fight, at least one of us needed to be present to support Cayden. Everyone I knew was either too scared of COVID or too busy or just didn't feel that strongly to want to go with me. So I picked up my black eye shadow and did what I had wanted to do all week. I painted my eye sockets with eye shadow and streaked them to look like tears. This was my war paint. This was a war on women, and I was preparing for battle. I also painted it to represent 'the sad one'—the part of me that had absorbed all of the trauma from Hope.

My hair braided back to expose the footprints for Hope, and the war paint was for me.

I am taking me back.

I repeated it out loud. The kids were shocked at my eye makeup, and I would later learn that two-year-old Ember tried to mimic me and colored her face with an orange marker. My little suffragette. Christopher helped me pack water and snacks for the end of the march and ensured I had the pepper gel spray he bought me in case someone attacked me over the sign.

No one would ever get the chance.

I parked at the end of the parade route and was mentally prepared to walk to the beginning because I was too broke as a joke for bus fare. I kept my eyes down as I left my car, my sign covered in my poncho, careful not to make eye contact. I looked at the center of the road where the streetcar station was. I crossed the street where other women who were clearly there for the march stood. I asked them how much it cost to ride and was relieved to hear it was free. I told them "thank you" because I was scared to walk alone, to which they replied that I could stick with them. I felt brave in their numbers and removed my poncho from the sign and stuffed it in my purse. Small gasps escaped their lips as they read it. One asked if that was my story, to which I replied in affirmation. She said, "Thank you for sharing. You are really very brave." She then took a picture of me with my sign.

The streetcar ride was far shorter than my attempt at trekking to the beginning would have been. Hundreds of women and a sprinkling of men met at the rendezvous point. Women of all walks, in all sorts of attire, and a wide specter of signs milled about the large parking lot. I was scared, so I stood just inside the parking lot, leaned my sign against me, and waited for the march to start.

It didn't take long for women to start approaching me, asking me about my sign. I explained about Hope's condition and why I took the option of abortion to save my life and end her suffering. Women cried with me, held their hands to their hearts, and embraced me—pandemic be damned. Each woman poured respect and love into me from their cup, and slowly I felt my own cup start to fill until it was spilling over with support. I stood up taller, and when it was time to start, I was near the front of the line, protected and surrounded by women. I did not need to fear, or feel shame, or guilt any longer.

It was a hot uphill walk, and when I stopped over to the side to catch my breath from my mask, two women in pink wigs with pink signs stopped and gave me water and waited with me until I was ready to rejoin the group. I was so deeply thankful for their help, and they helped me dig deeper to find the strength to finish the march. A woman even stopped me on the march because she had been through the same thing I did and was so proud of me for standing up for women like us.

When we got to the end, I found myself standing next to the stage where the speaker was. One by one, people came up to embrace me, literally and figuratively, and took pictures to share and so they could find my story on my website. The speakers moved me to tears. The talk about abortion and birth control being essential healthcare rang out to me, and I held up my sign a little higher. A female pastor even shared about her rape survival and abortion story. I knew that if she could stand up for herself at that moment, I could do it for Hope and me.

I returned home after the rally, showered, and cuddled with Ember, trying to get her to take a nap to no avail. I was tired, but my soul was energized. That night, there was a special concert as a continuation of the rally. I had front row tickets because they were highly affordable, and there was just a small group going.

It was in a church that I had been skeptical about. I hadn't set foot in a church with other people doing church things in it in a very long time. I parked my car and walked up to the stairs. Before I walked up the stairs, a woman stopped me to tell me how brave I was for my sign and that she loved my eye makeup. I told her, "thank you," and handed her a flyer with my information on it and explained a little about my story. She was excited to check it out. I looked up the concrete steps and saw the pastor from the rally. I was scared, but I introduced myself and thanked her for telling her story. I told her that it inspired me to share my story, and I told her about Hope, and she embraced me. She then gave me her card to help me find a home church or if I needed to talk, and I gave her a flyer, before she took a picture of it for safekeeping.

The music artist, Summer, was standing outside the church now. I caught her on her way in and thanked her for her music at the rally as it moved me to tears and shared my story about Hope. She recognized me from the rally, hugged me, and told me that she would keep me in her prayers and meditation. I asked her if it was okay for me to hand out my flyers at her concert, to which she told me, "Of course."

A man checked my ticket, and I walked to the front of the church where took my seat. I was so scared of the church and of handing out my flyer that my knees were shaking. Soon, two men sat next to me. They were friendly and struck up the conversation, and one even noticed the flyers in my hands. He asked, "What do you get there?" I told them Hope and I's story and that I had permission to spread the word by handing the flyers out, but I was too nervous. He had me hand him the stack of flyers, and he split them between him and his friend. He then led me to the man who was the pastor of the church, explained what was going on, and the pastor asked if I wanted to tell my story to the audience. I froze but said yes. They led me to the stage of the church and gave me a microphone. I was shaking— my body and my voice. I had spoken in front of people for work all the time, but this was different. I was telling *our* story. This was vulnerable. This was scary.

I took a deep breath and said hello to the crowd. Everyone immediately stopped talking and turned their attention to me. I told them my name and said they might have seen me at the march with a black and white sign. I then explained our story, and when I finished, people stood and clapped for me.

I had taken *me* back.

The night of the rally, while I slept, I met 'the sad one' in my dreams. Her eyes were not nearly as dark, her skin not as ghastly pale. She and I met at a river. We sat in the babbling water. She let me wash the evidence of the storm away. I took a sponge and wiped away the sand from her mouth, the blood from her eyes, and her neck. I brushed her long black hair and pulled it away from her face.

I sat beside her, and in the reflection of the soft current, the sad one was replaced by Philmont Kelsey, but older, and more assured in herself. It wasn't long before I realized that the reflection looking back at me was my own.

I had taken *me* back.